Color Your Stress Away

GEOMETRICAL PATTERNS

COLORING BOOK FOR ADULTS
WITH INSPIRING ART QUOTES

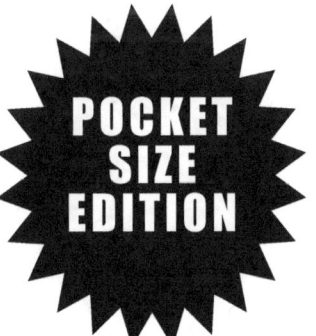

POCKET SIZE EDITION

Marie-Judith Jean-Louis

THE PURPOSE OF ART IS WASHING AWAY THE DUST OF DAILY LIFE OFF OUR SOULS.

PABLO PICASSO

How to Color Your Stress Away

Remember when you used to color as a kid? You just picked up a pencil and filled in the pages however you wanted. You didn't worry about anything, you weren't overwhelmed by your thoughts, you were just enjoying coloring. Turns out coloring is one of the easiest, most affordable and effective way to give your mind a break, wether you're getting ready to go to bed, on vacation or during a lunch break. There are no rules when it comes to coloring for adults, just go with what feels good to you in the moment. Just pick up a couple pencils and bring the pages to life. Don't worry about matching colors or even finishing the pages. Let your subconscious guide you to release your stress and replenish your energy.

Coloring is the new meditation, yoga for the brain. Take a couple minutes everyday to add some color and you should notice the difference in the way you feel even after one session. Coloring is known to not only help reduce stress but also to increase productivity, to help with depression, to help you sleep better, and to make you feel better.

Reconnect with your inner child. Let you creativity grow and if you feel inclined to, share your sketches on Facebook and Instagram with the #coloryourstressaway.

Happy coloring!
MJ

I DON'T LISTEN TO WHAT ART CRITICS SAY. I DON'T KNOW ANYBODY WHO NEEDS A CRITIC TO FIND OUT WHAT ART IS.

JEAN-MICHEL BASQUIAT

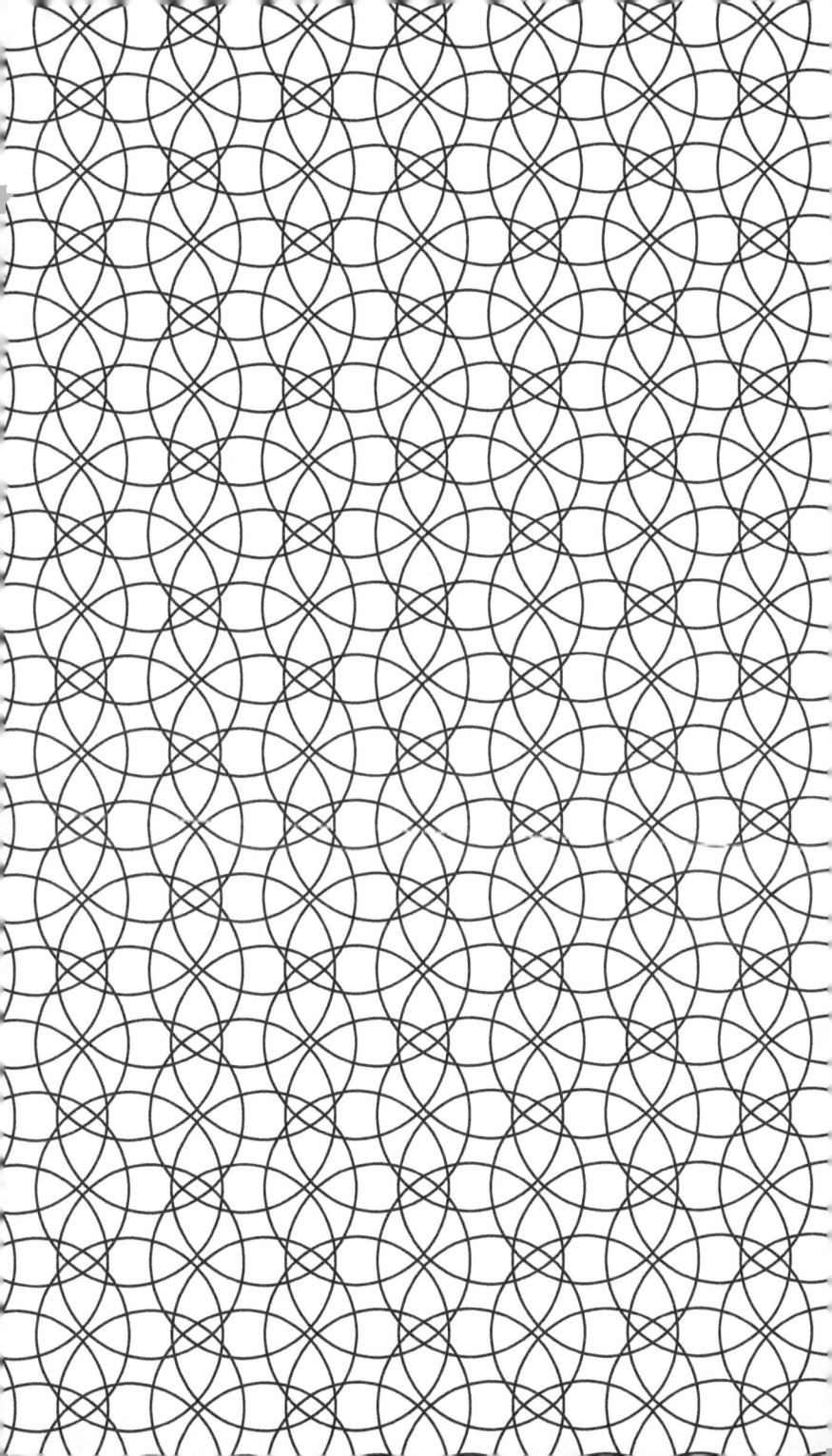

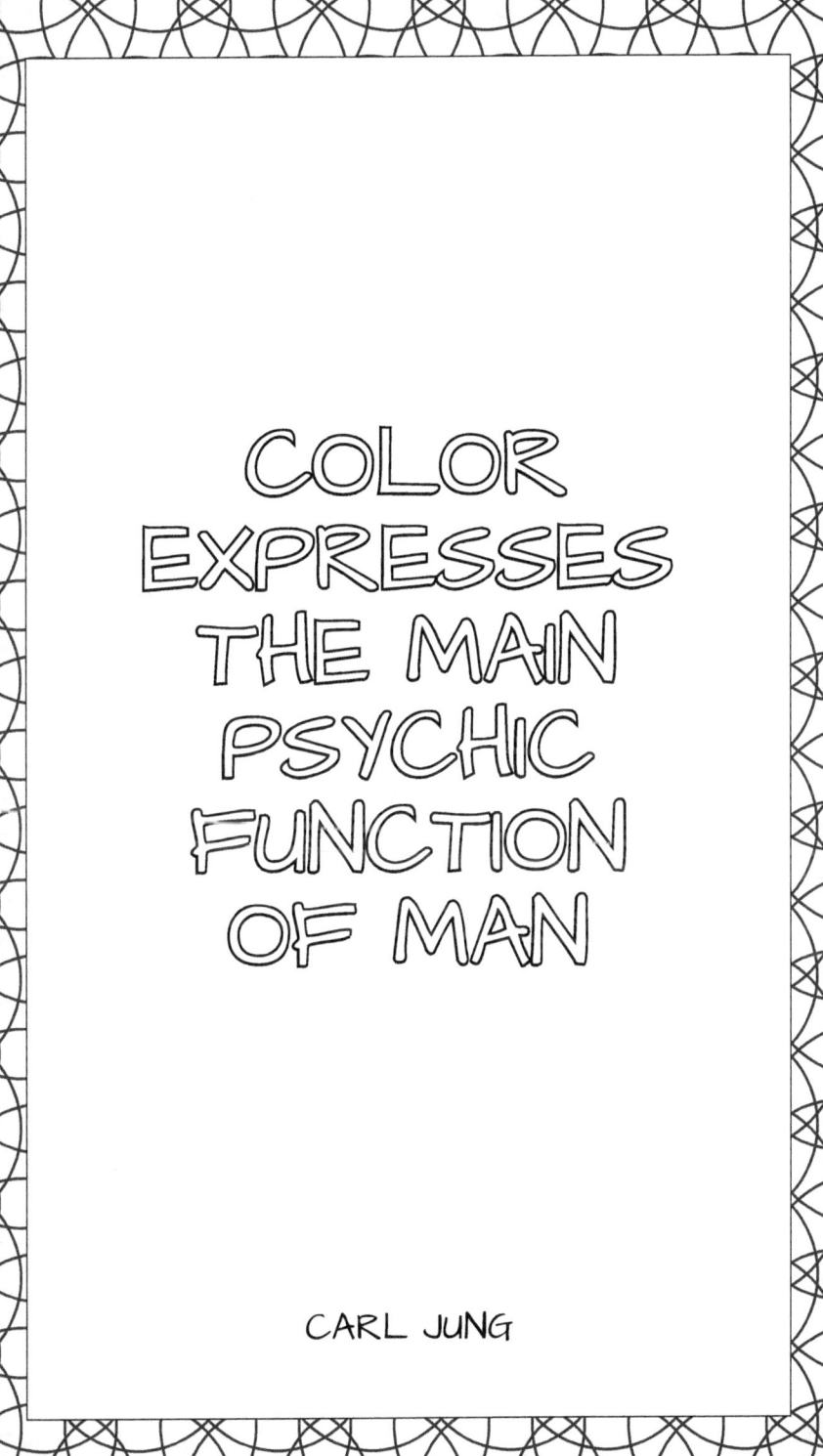

COLOR
EXPRESSES
THE MAIN
PSYCHIC
FUNCTION
OF MAN

CARL JUNG

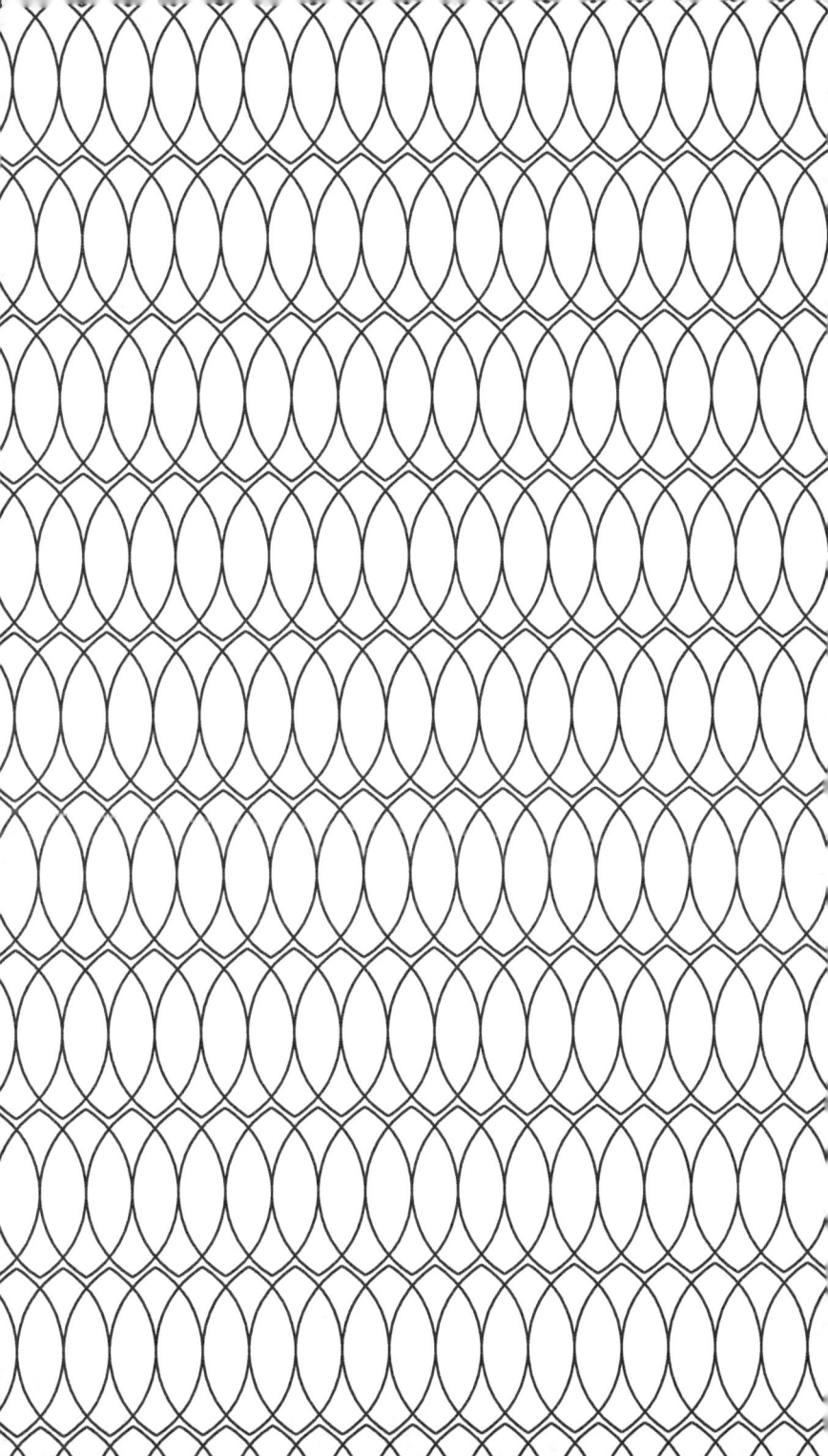

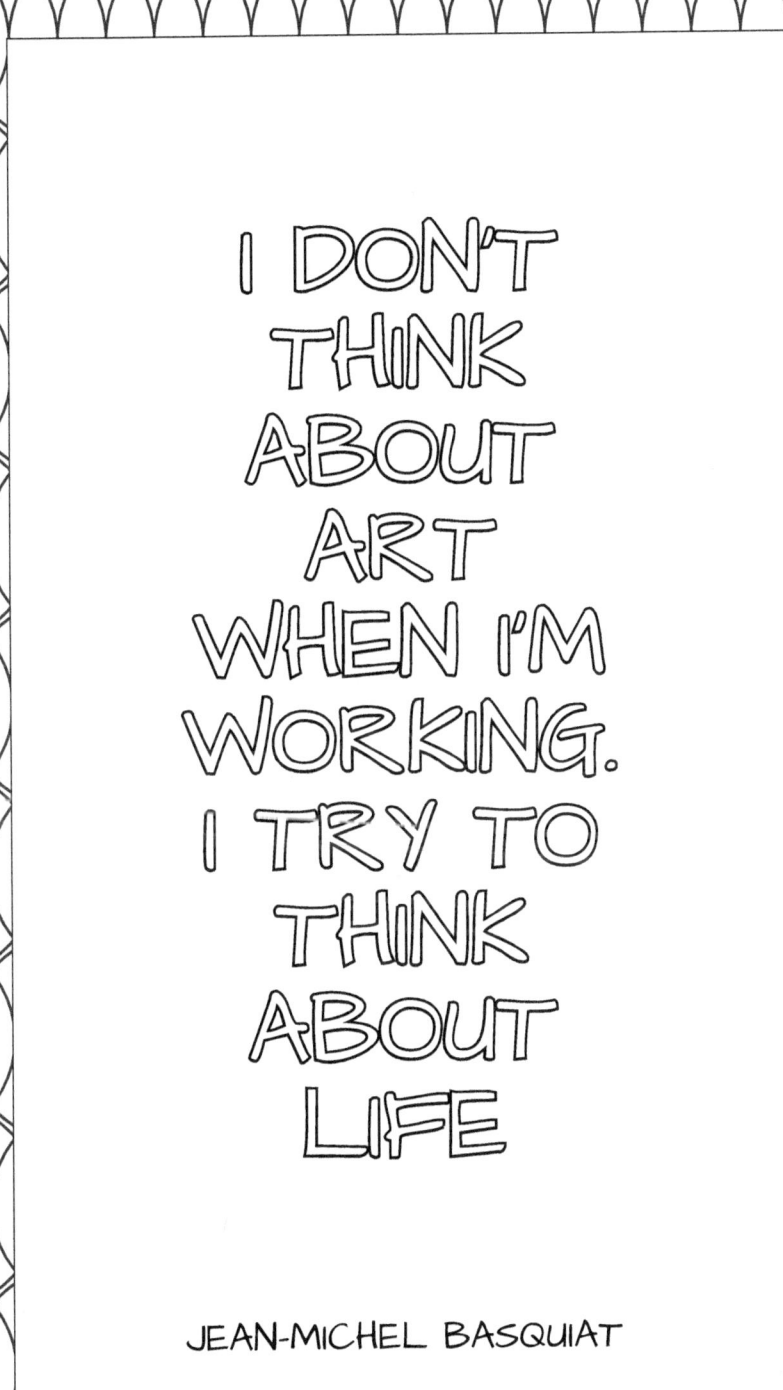

I DON'T THINK ABOUT ART WHEN I'M WORKING. I TRY TO THINK ABOUT LIFE

JEAN-MICHEL BASQUIAT

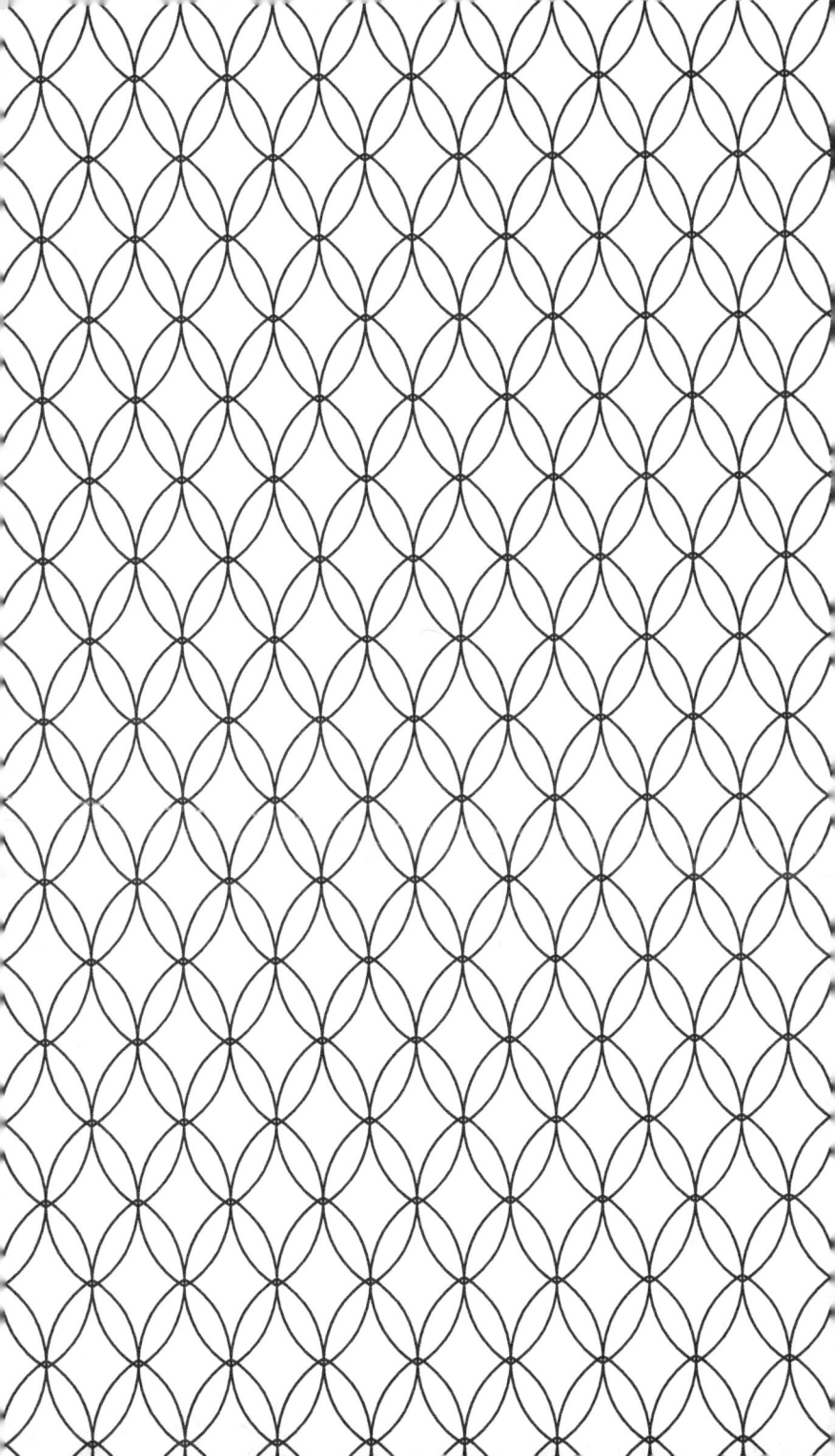

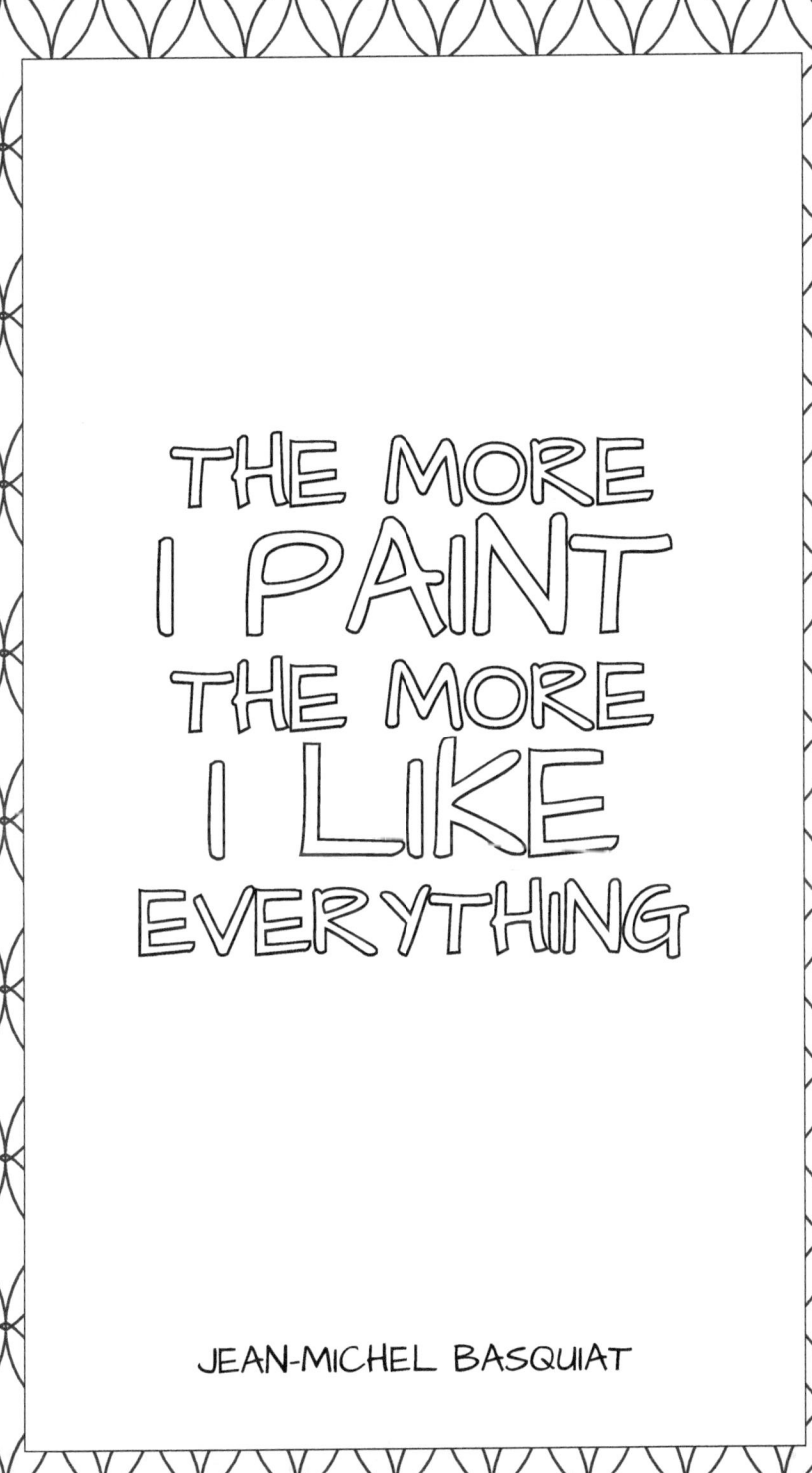

THE MORE
I PAINT
THE MORE
I LIKE
EVERYTHING

JEAN-MICHEL BASQUIAT

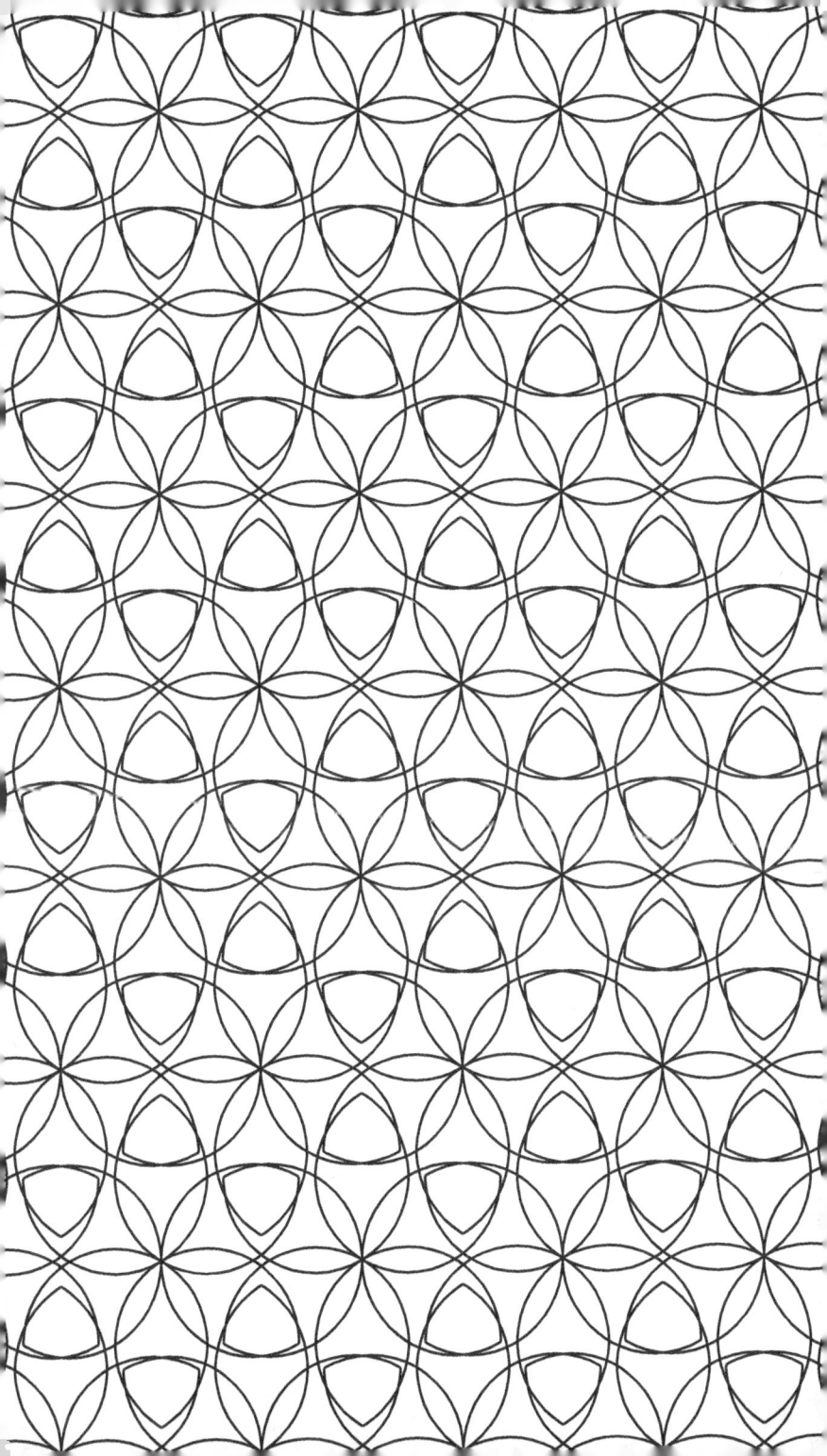

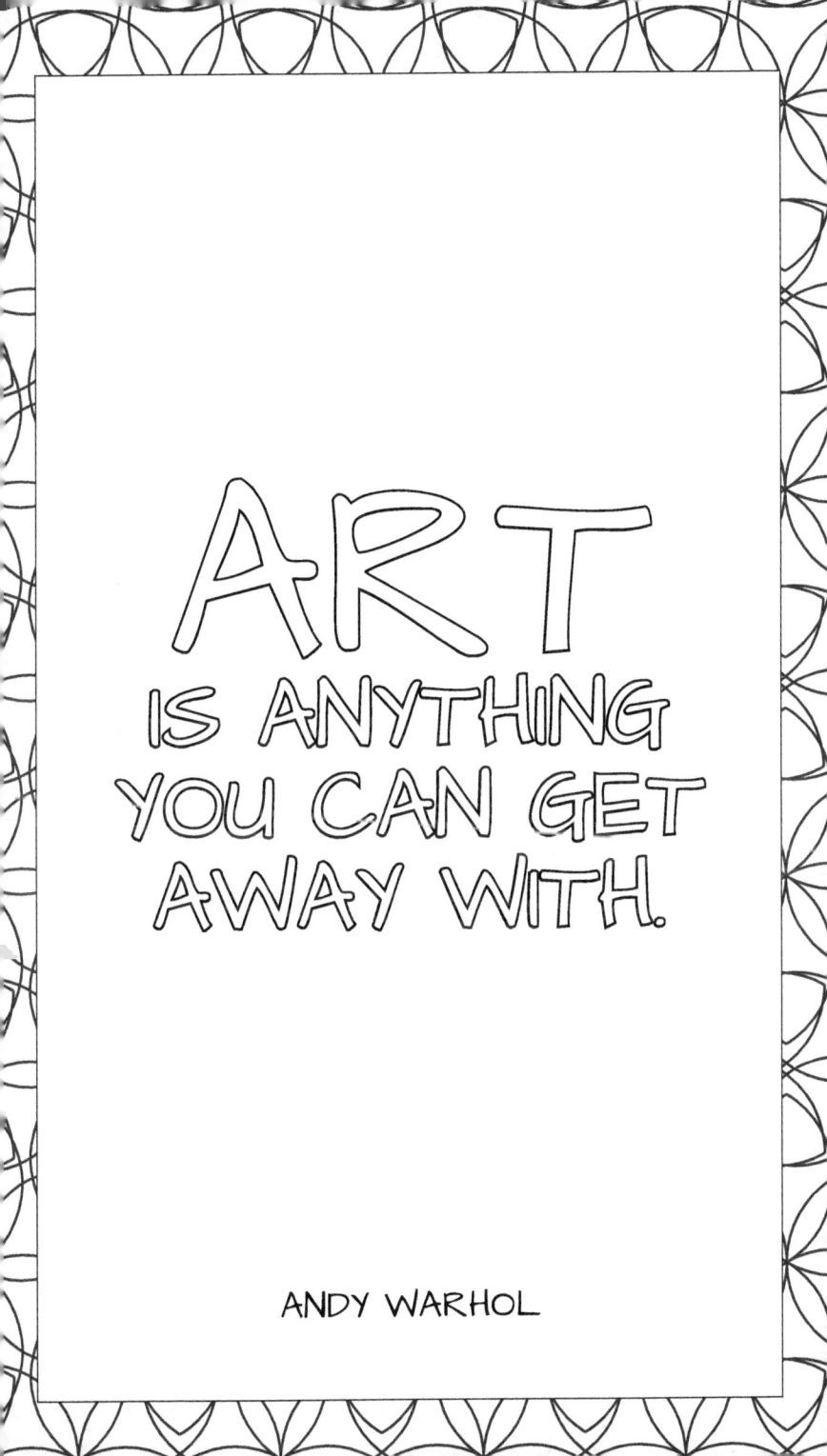

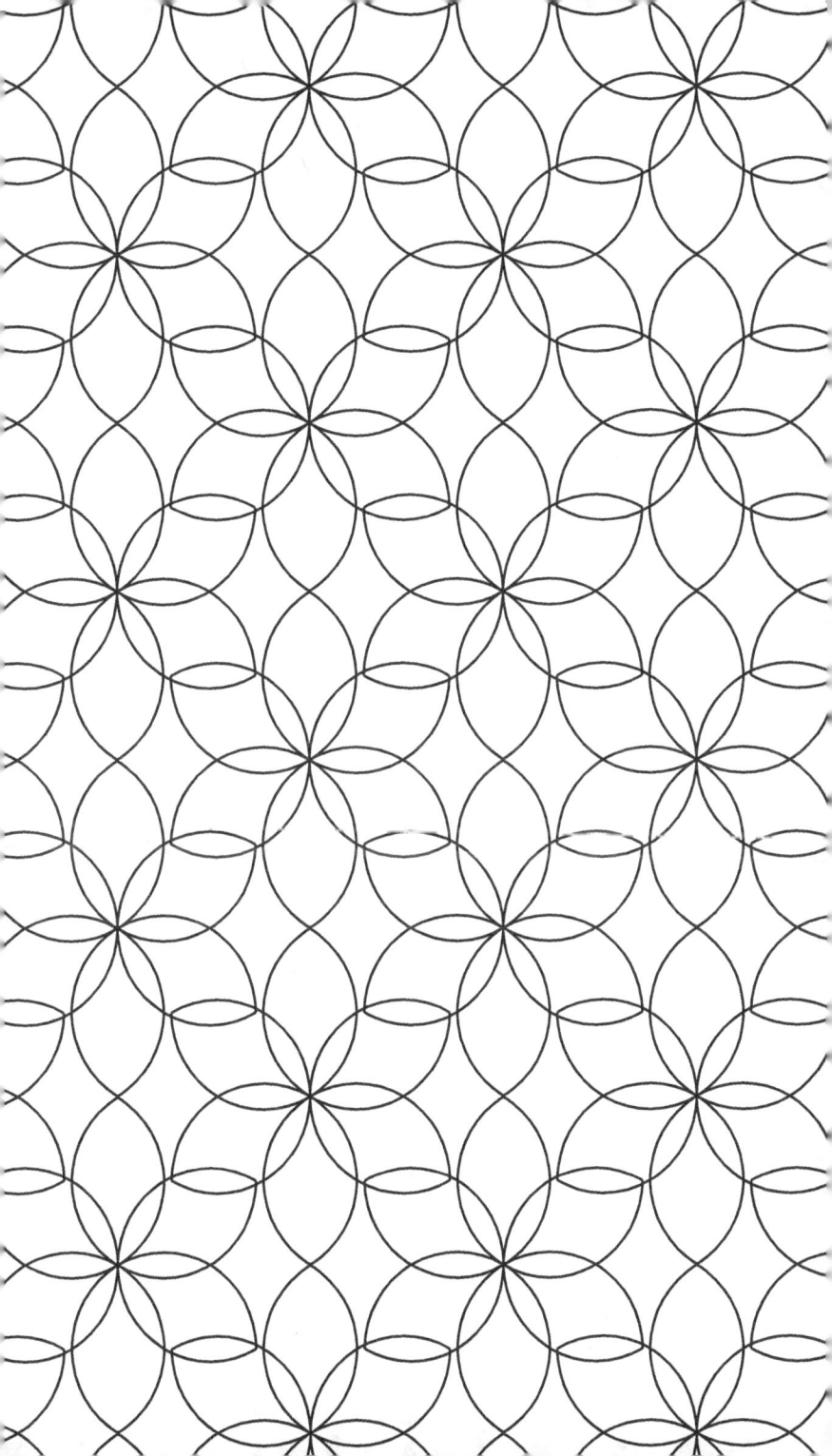

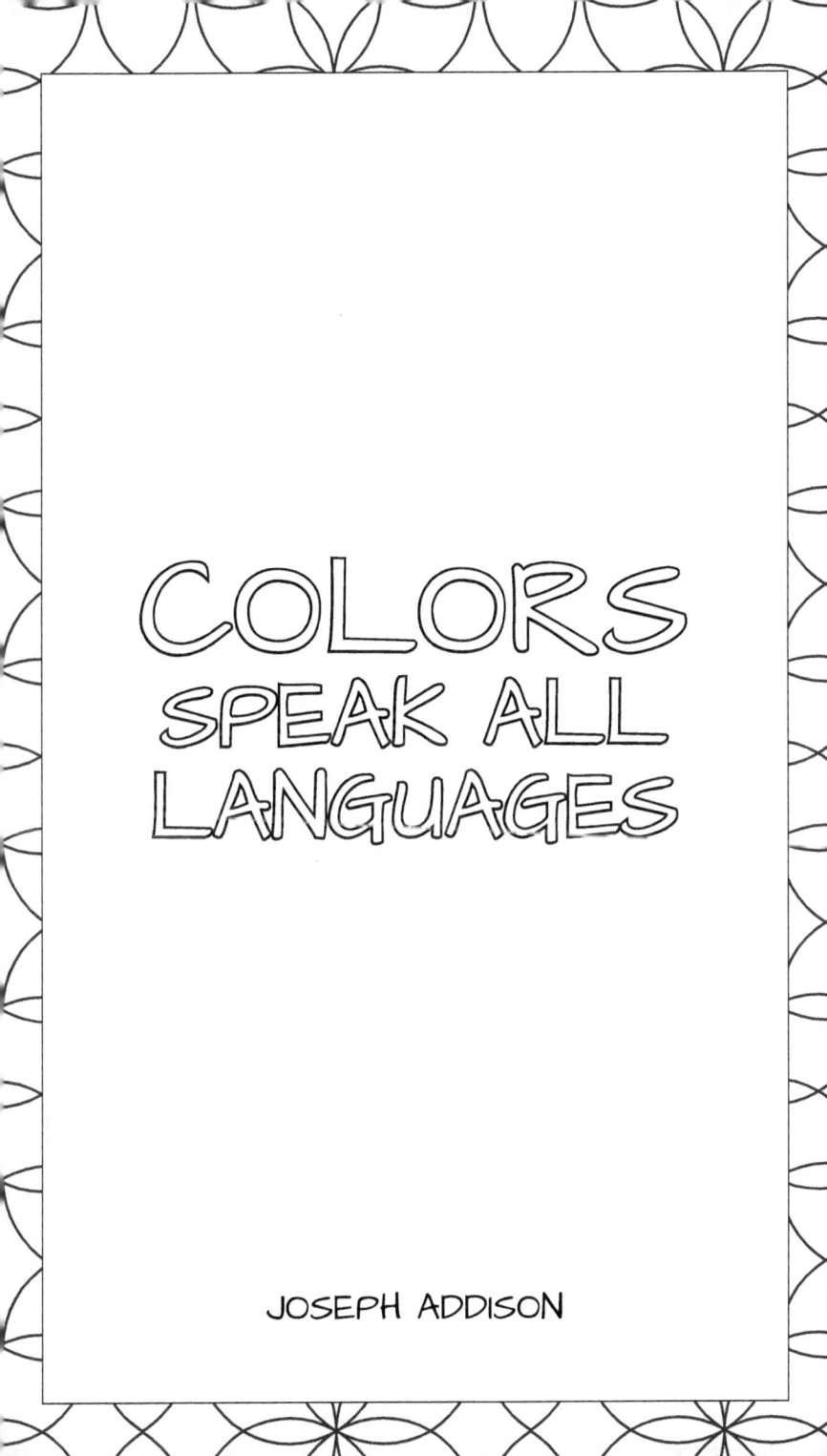

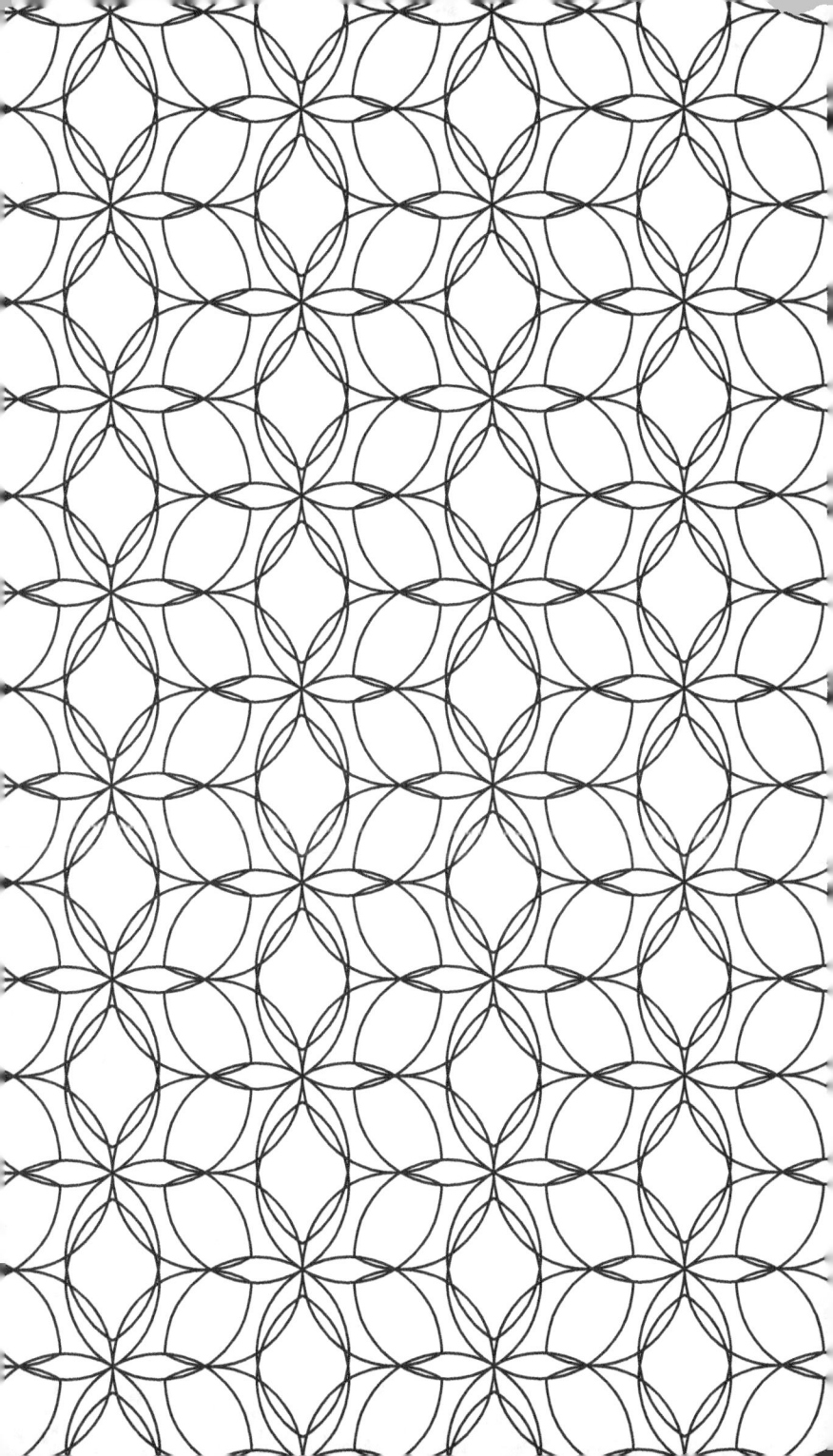

EVERYTHING HAS ITS BEAUTY BUT NOT EVERYONE SEES IT

ANDY WARHOL

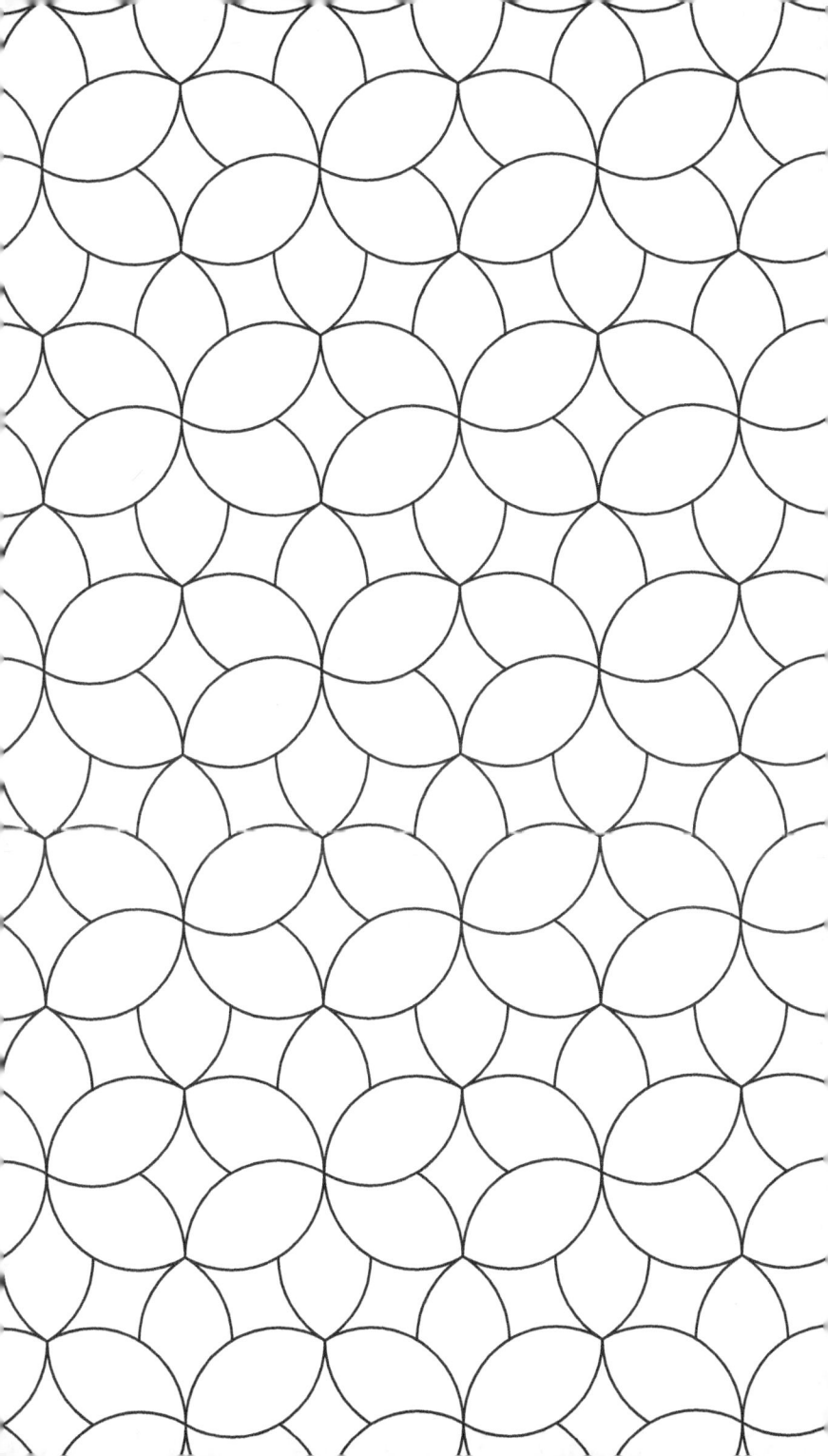

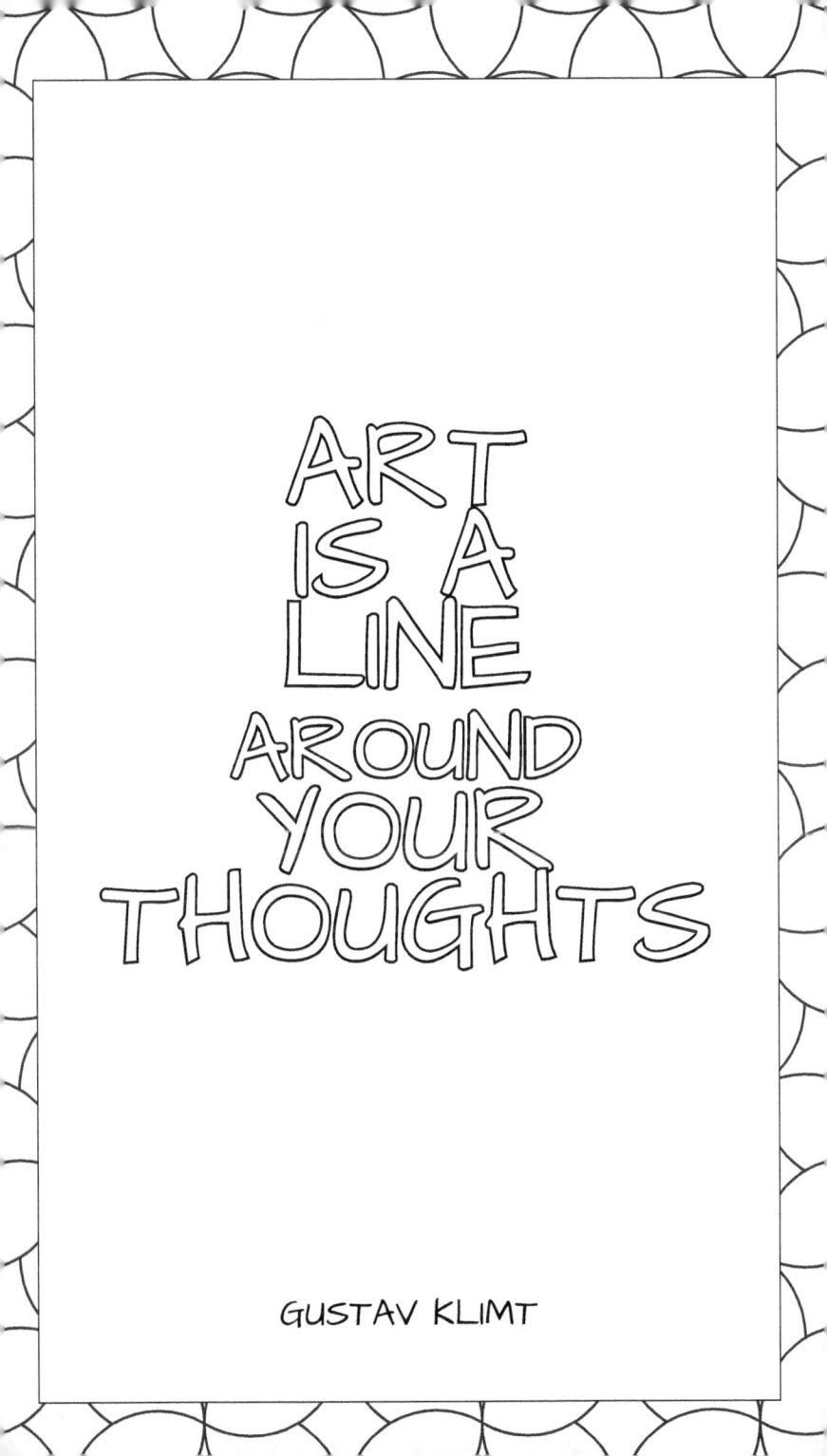

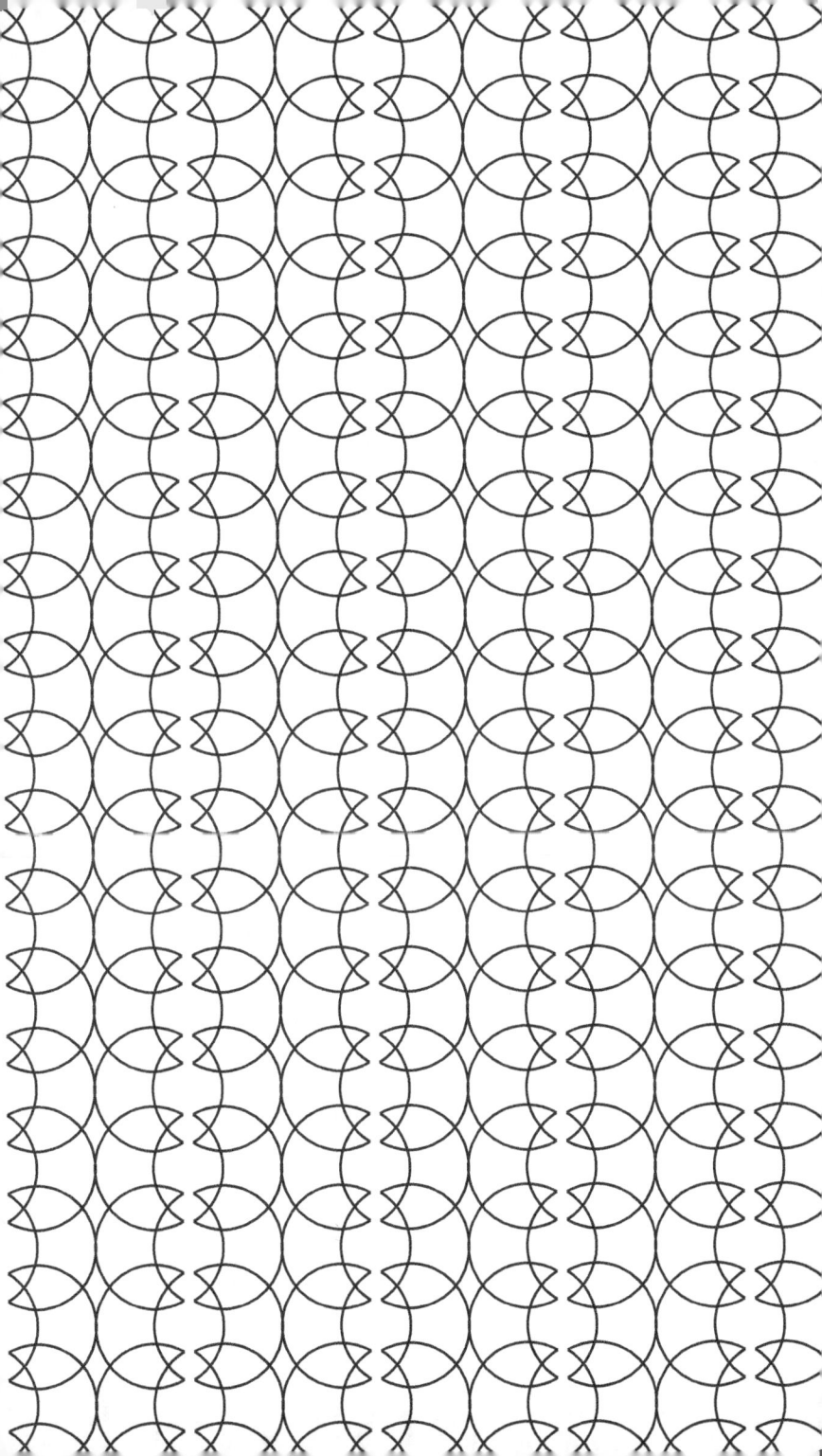

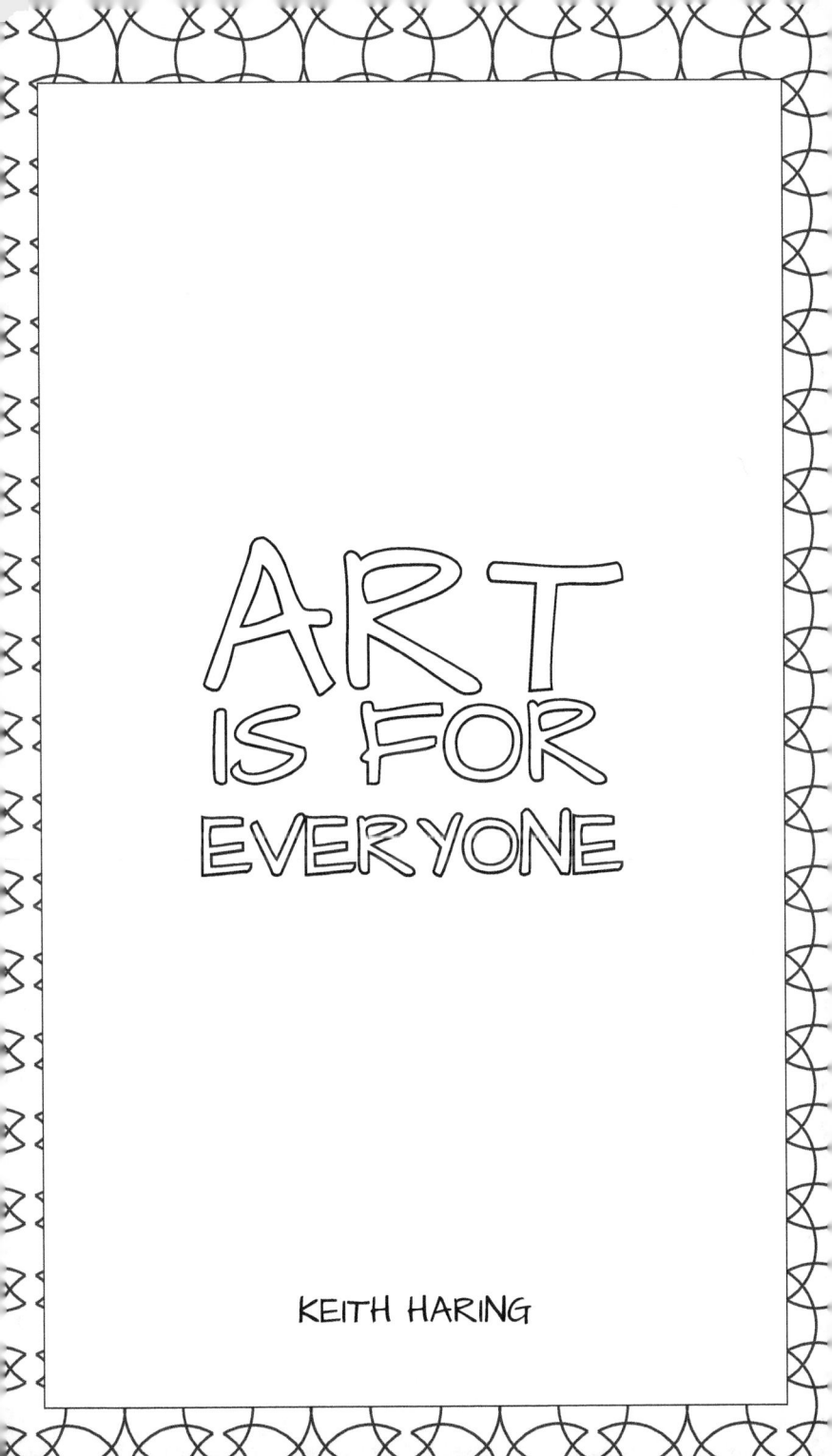

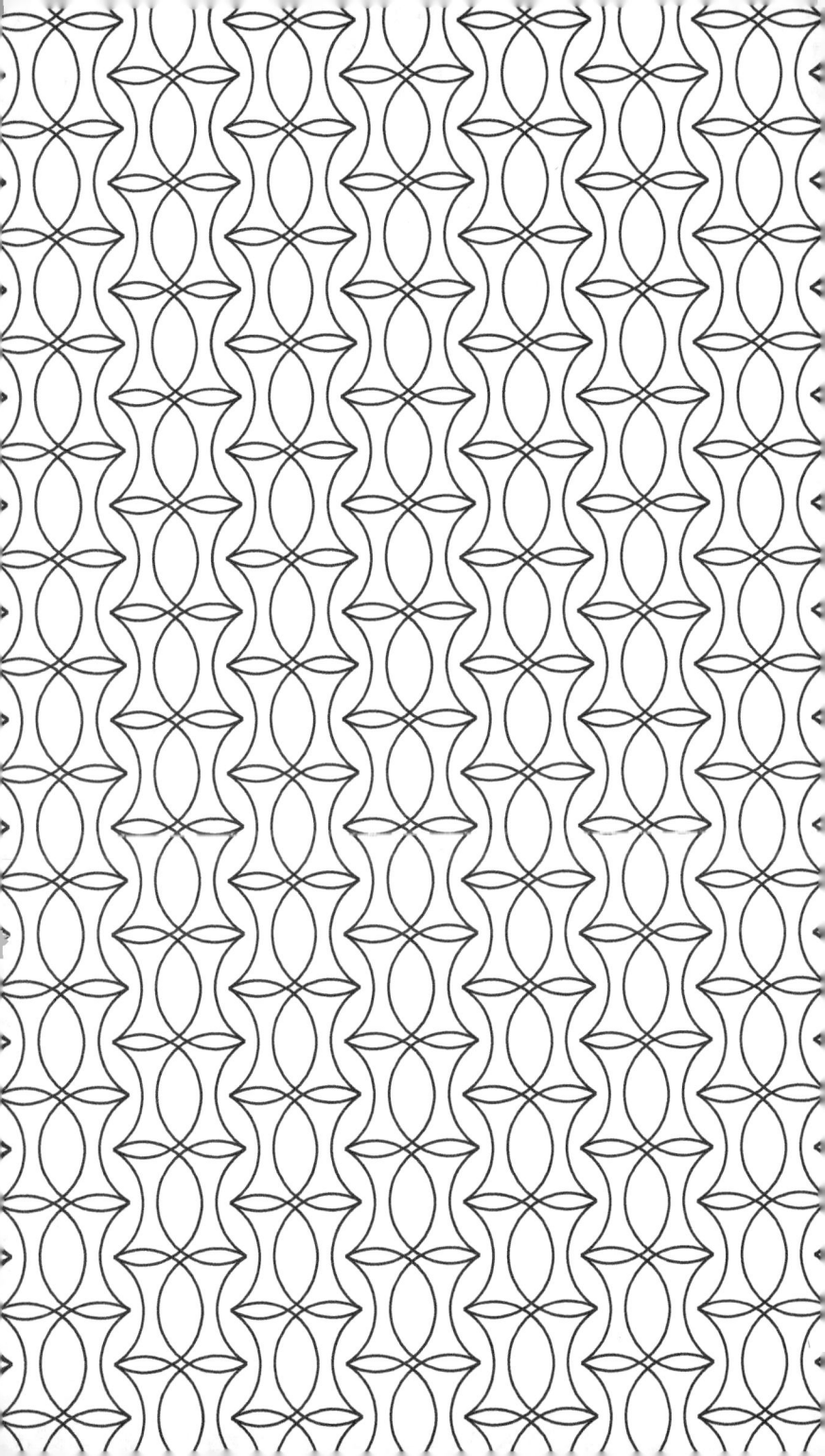

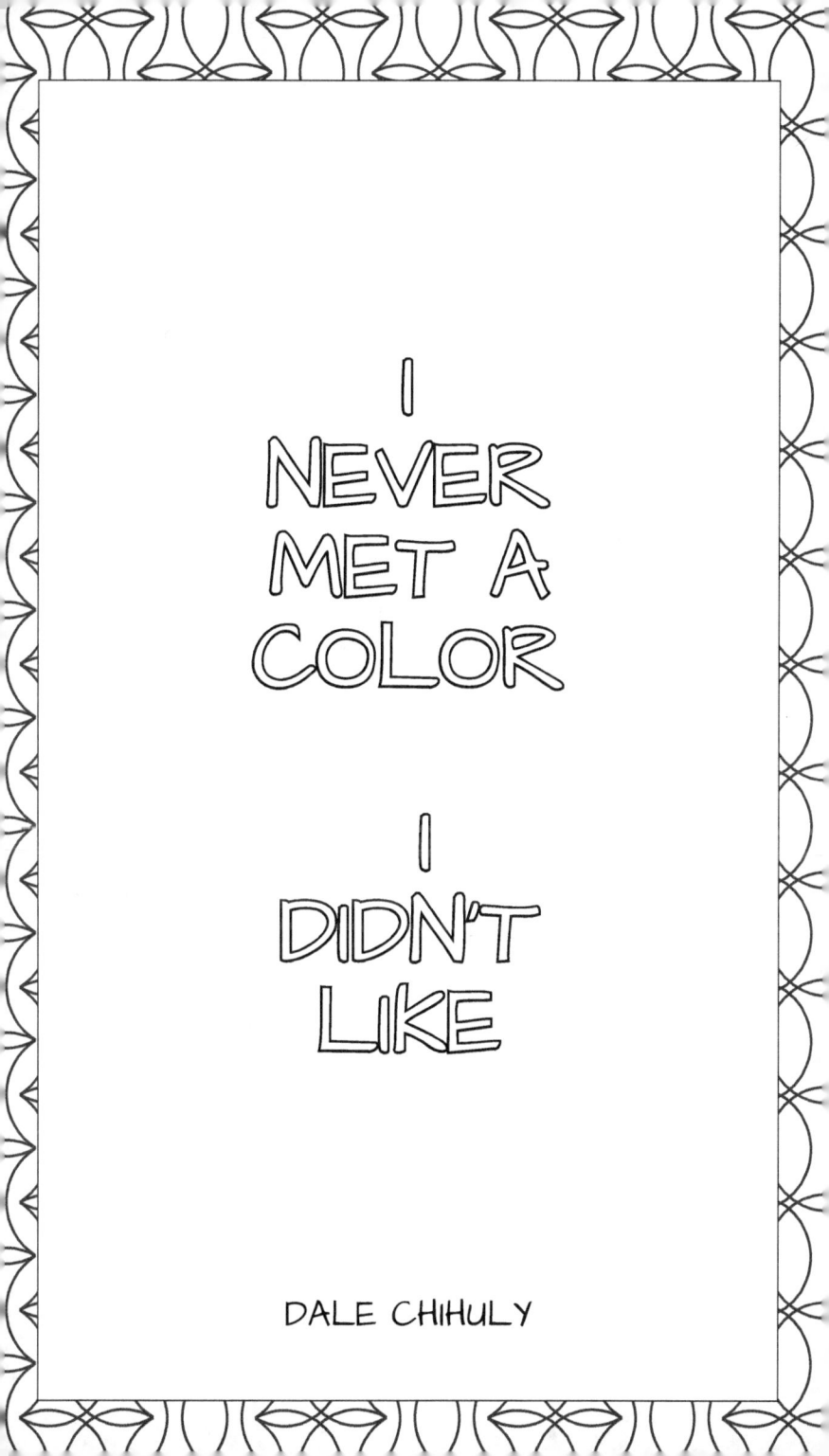

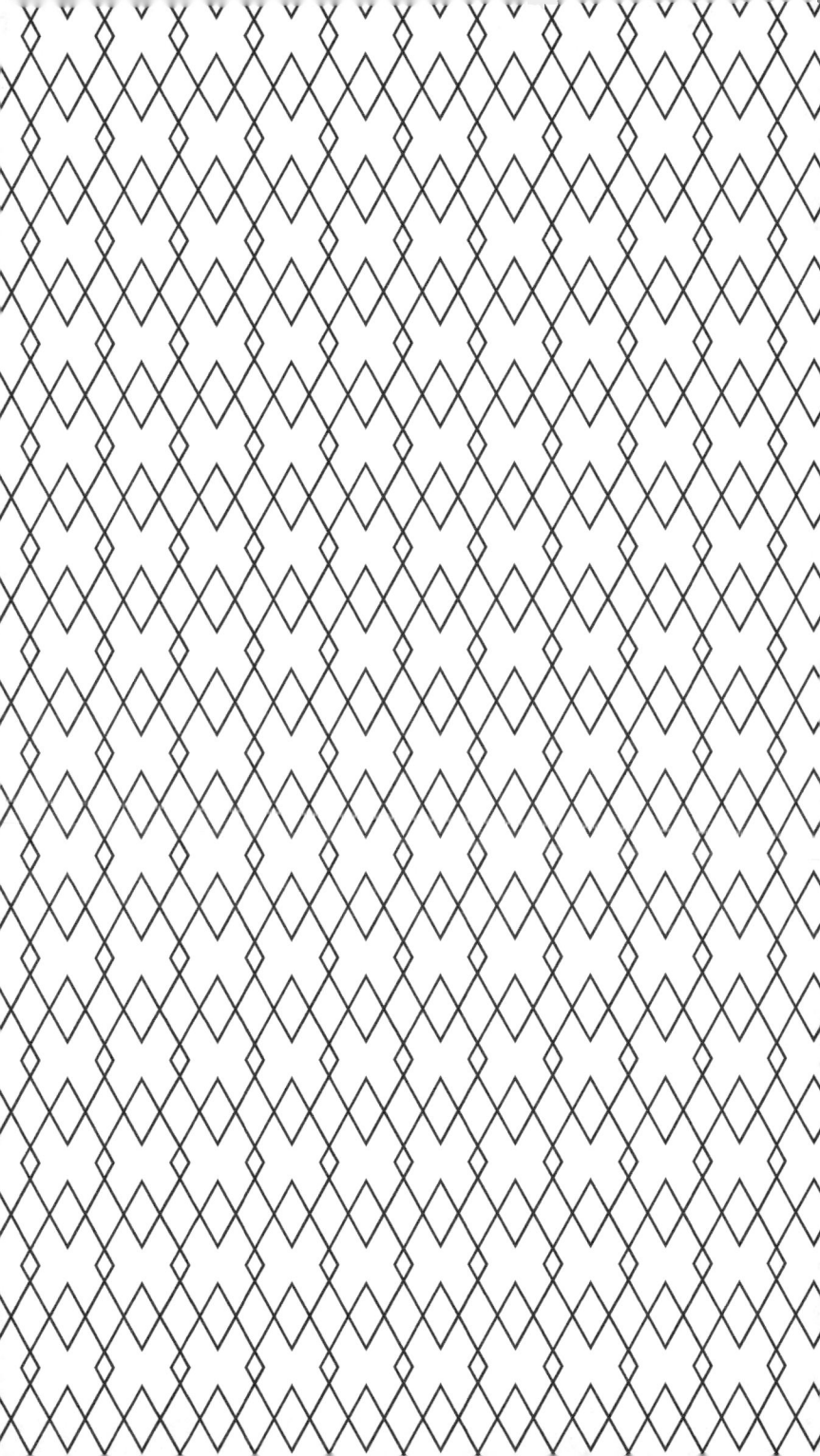

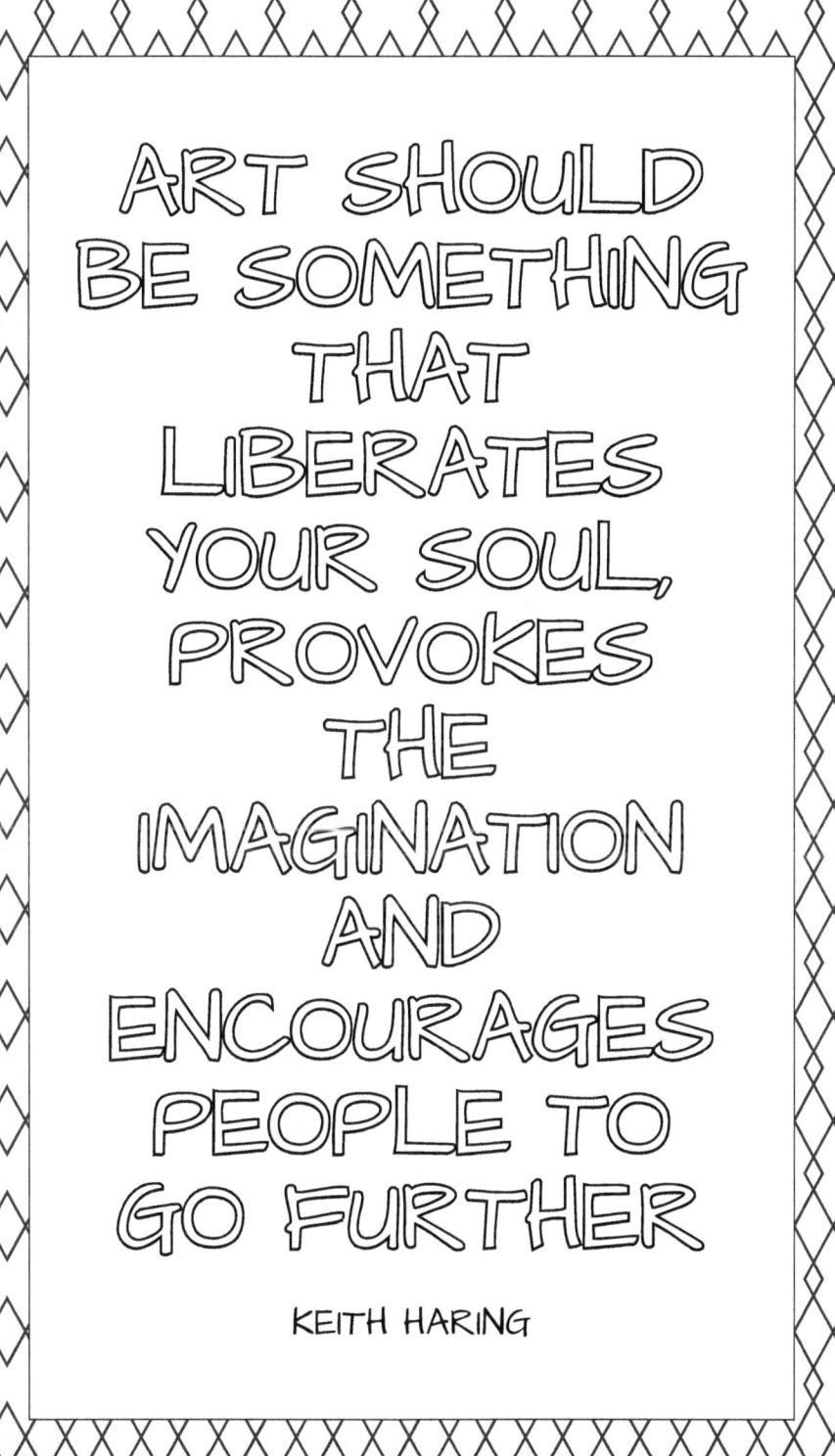

ART SHOULD BE SOMETHING THAT LIBERATES YOUR SOUL, PROVOKES THE IMAGINATION AND ENCOURAGES PEOPLE TO GO FURTHER

KEITH HARING

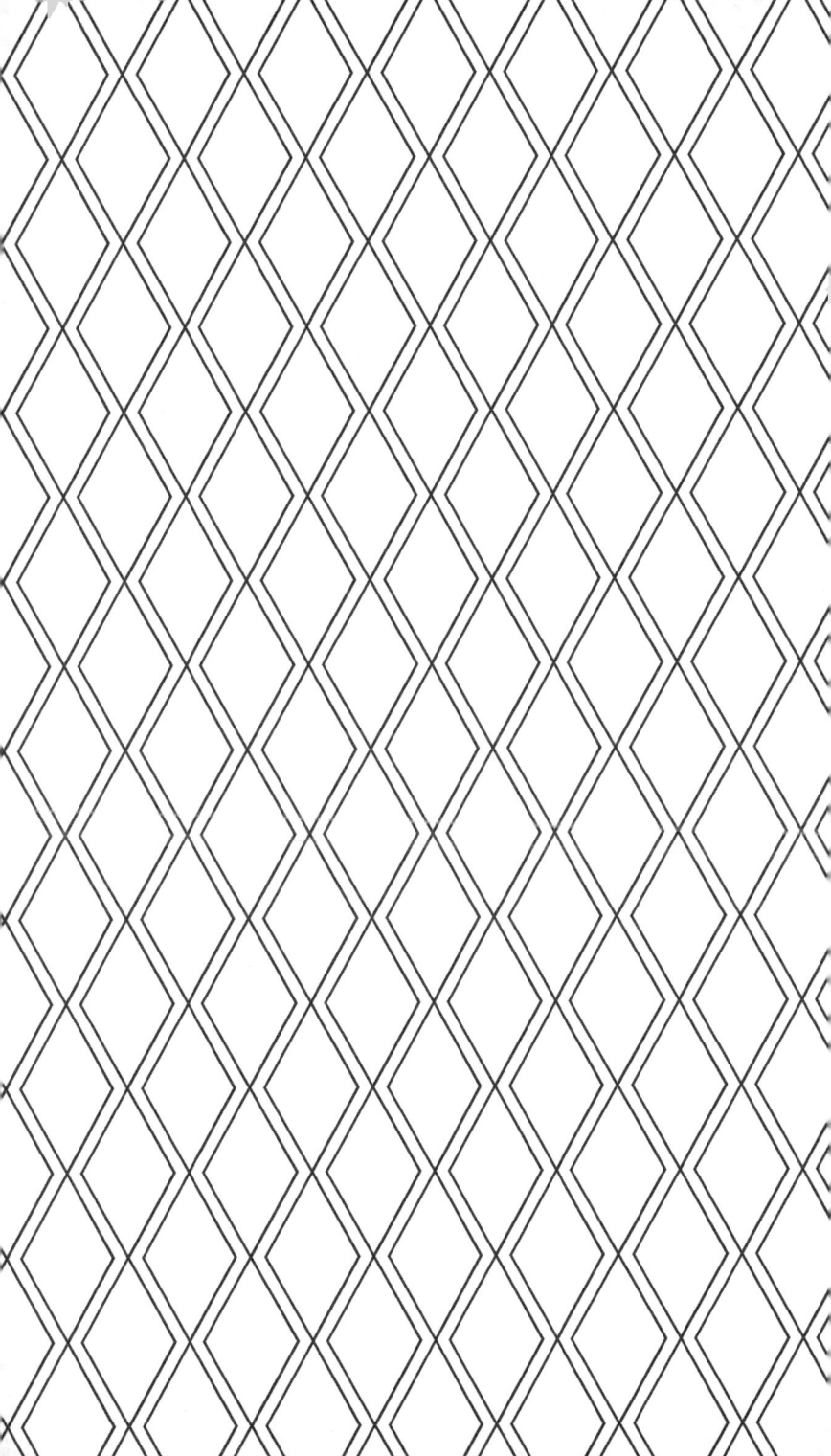

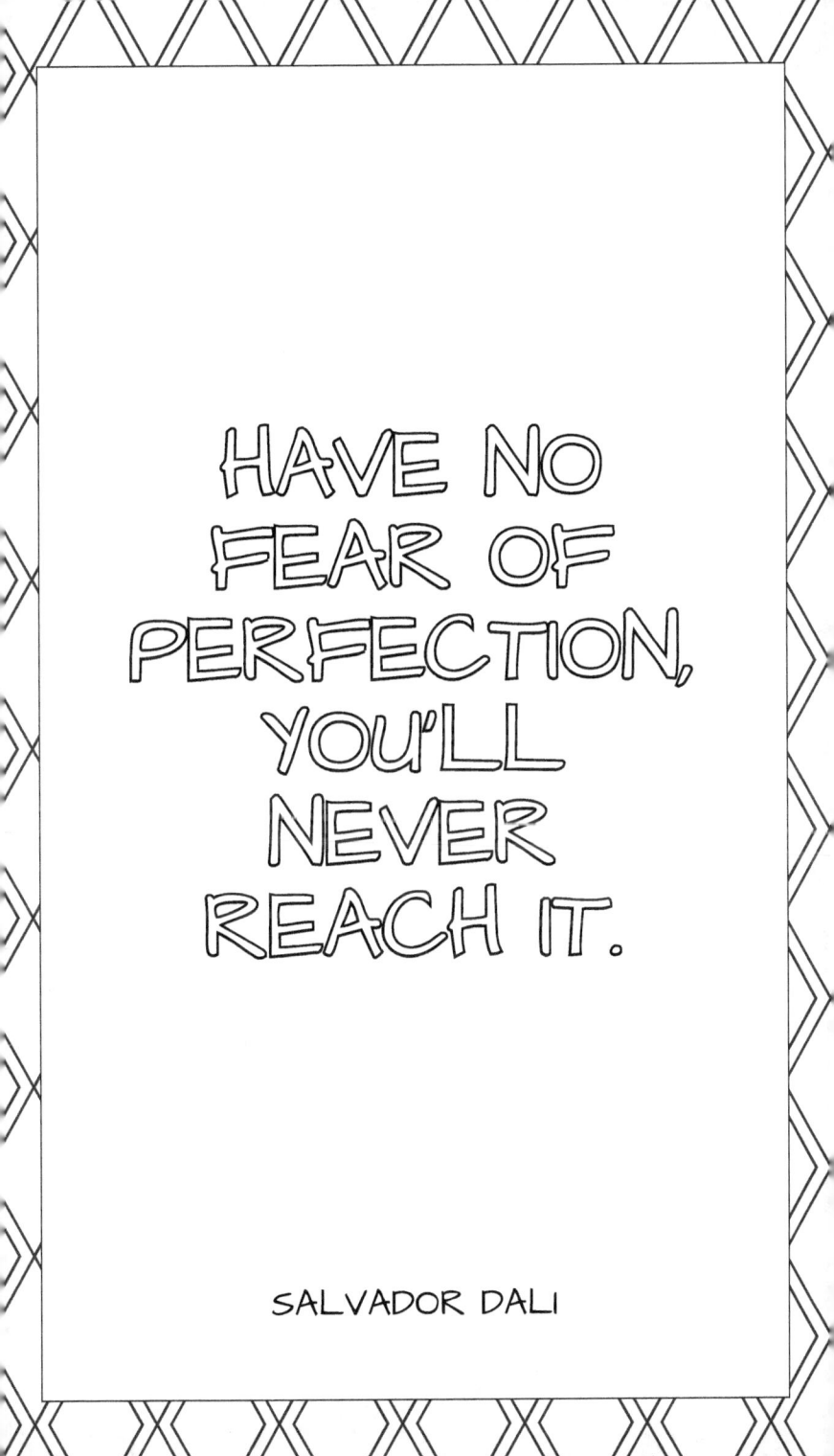

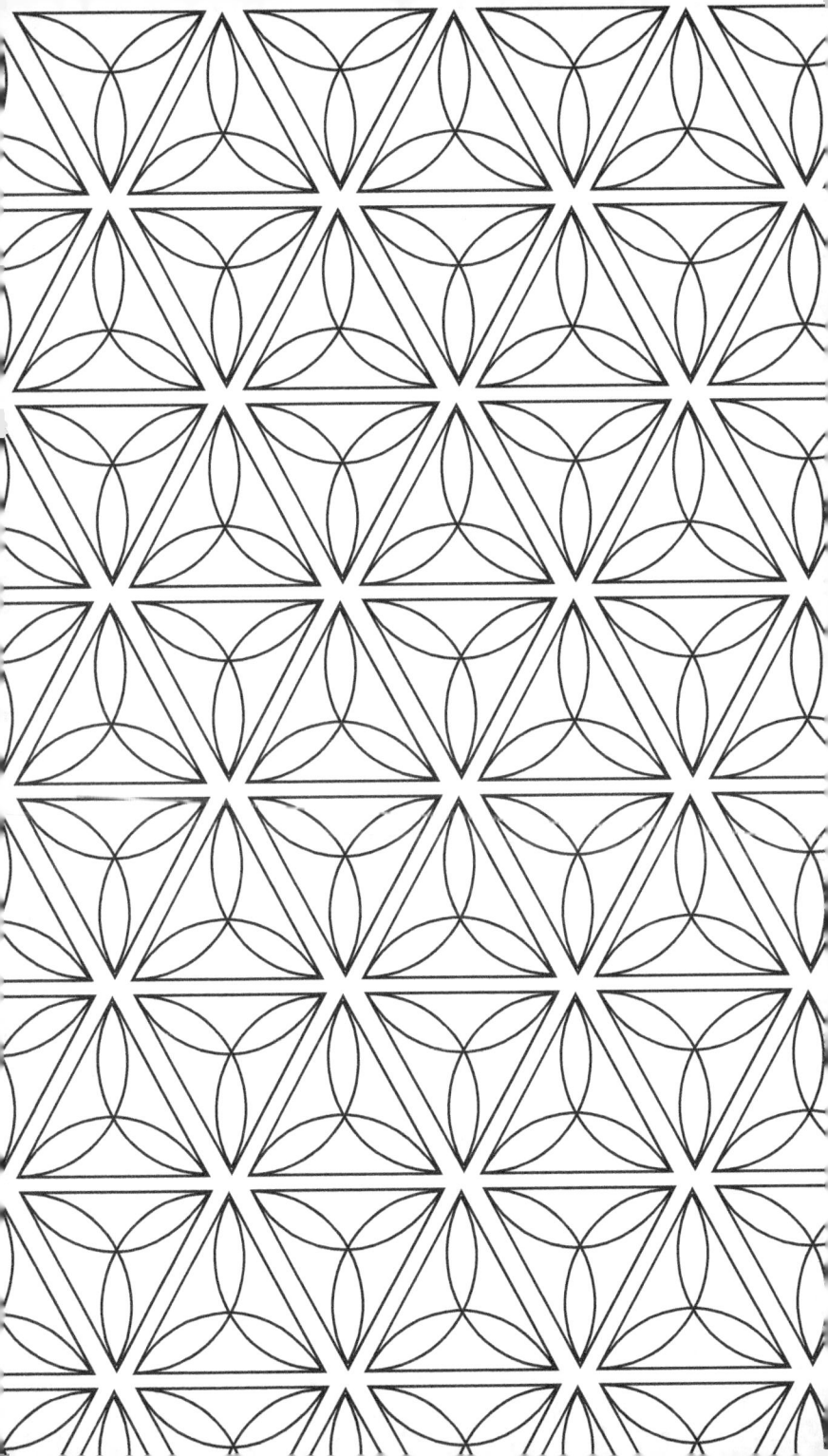

IT DOESN'T MATTER HOW PAINT IS PUT AS LONG AS SOMETHING IS SAID.

JACKSON POLLOCK

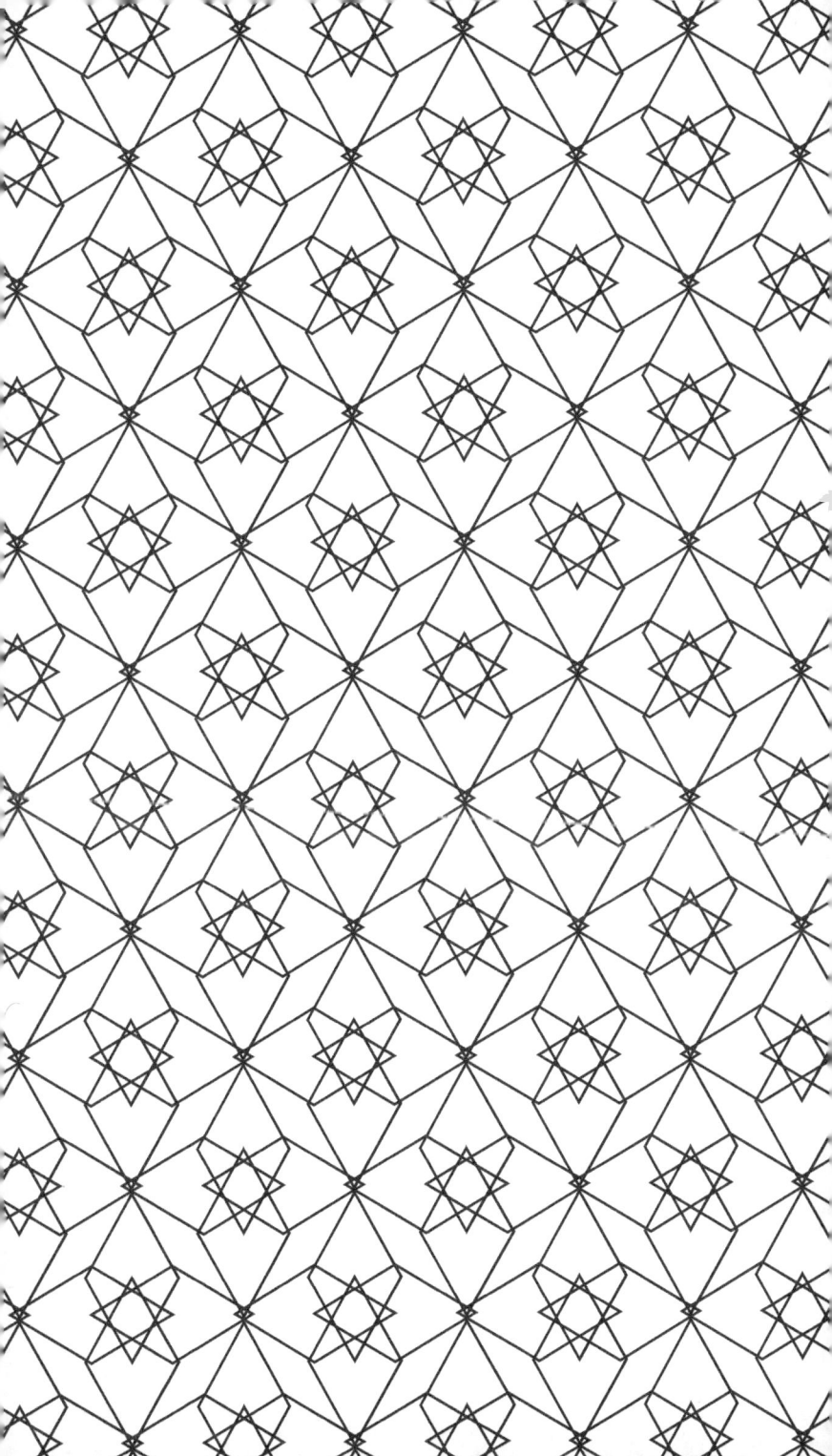

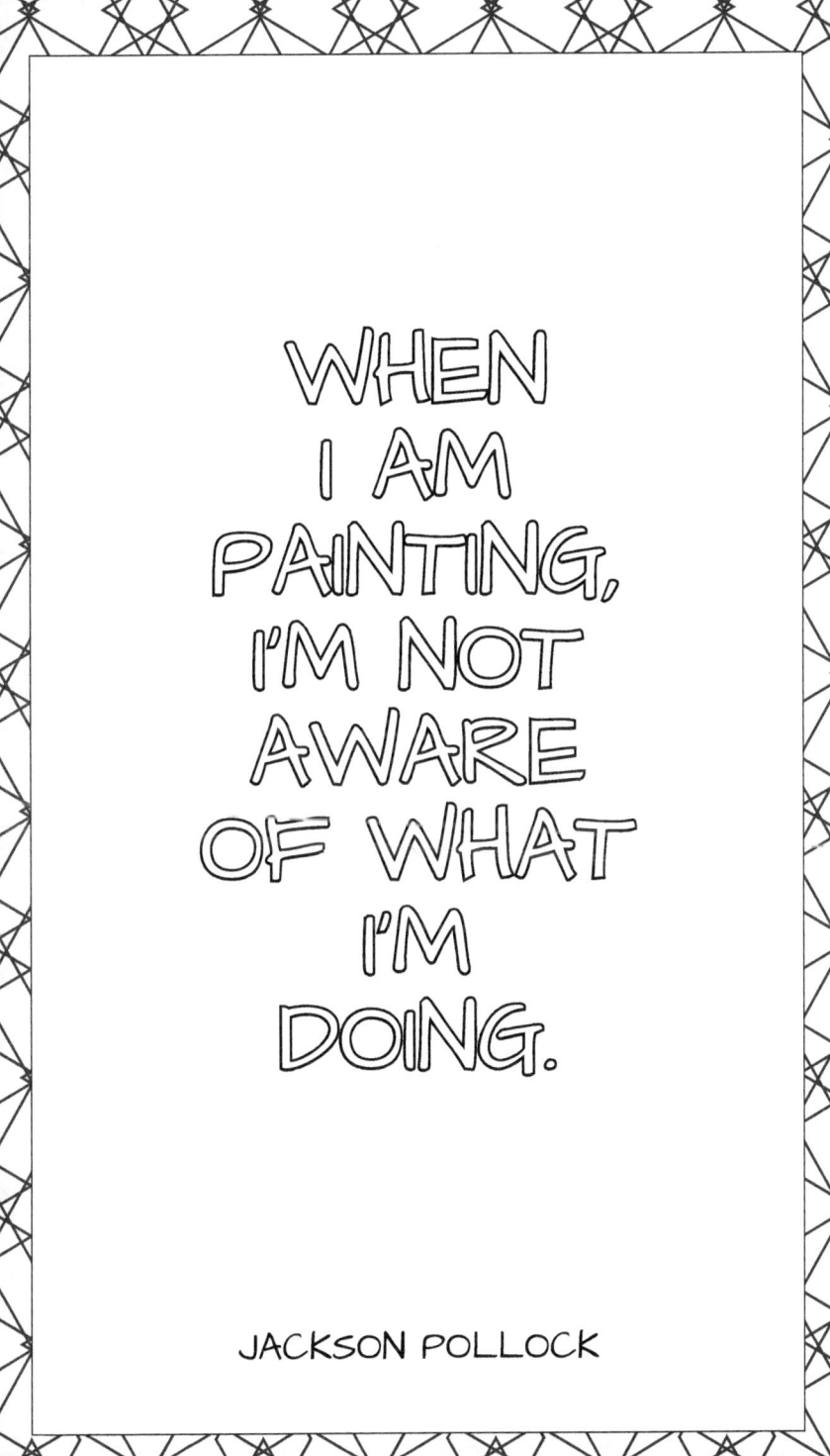

WHEN I AM PAINTING, I'M NOT AWARE OF WHAT I'M DOING.

JACKSON POLLOCK

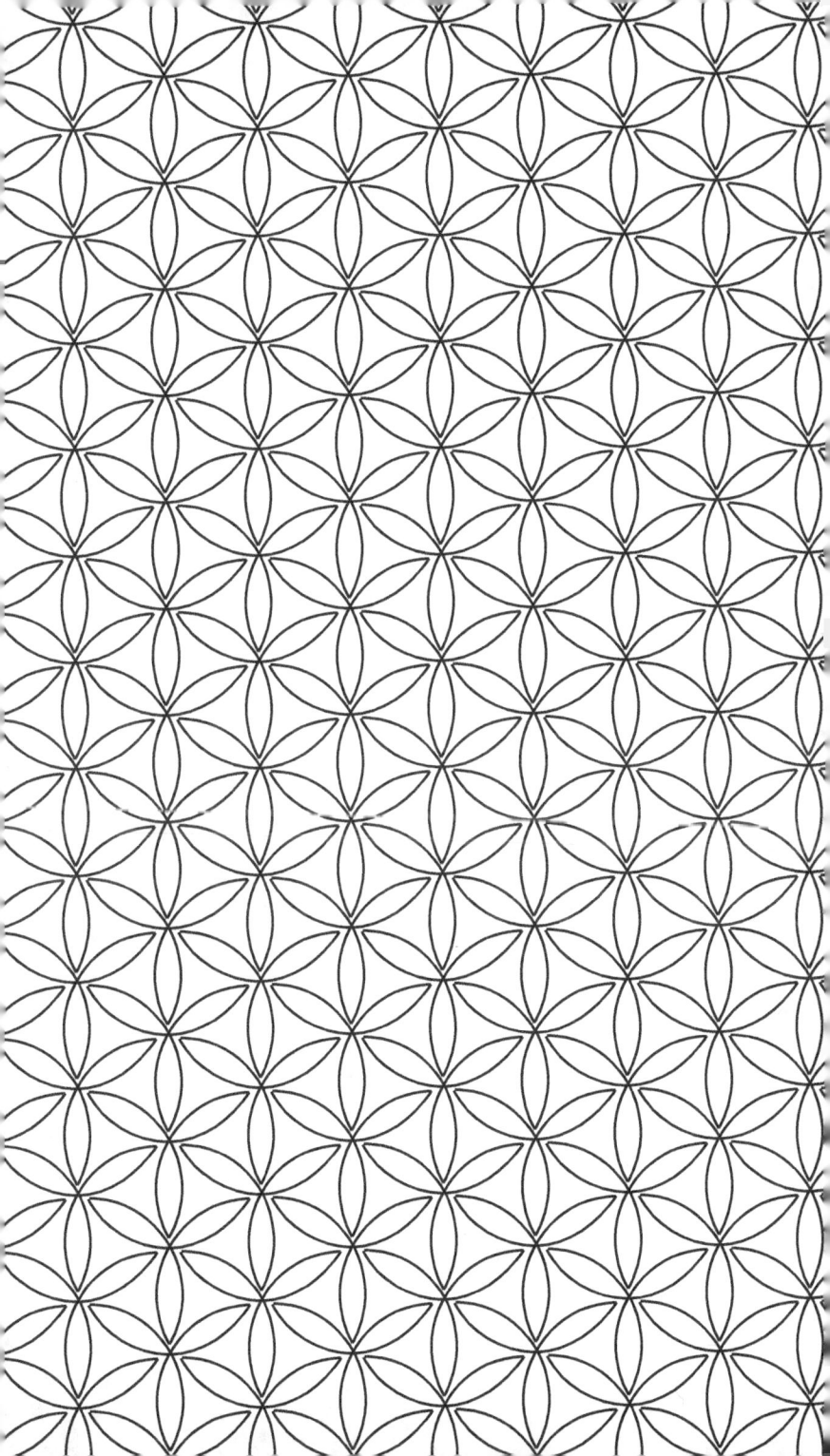

CREATIVE PEOPLE ARE CURIOUS, FLEXIBLE, PERSISTENT AND INDEPENDENT WITH A TREMENDOUS SPIRIT OF ADVENTURE AND A LOVE OF PLAY.

HENRI MATISSE

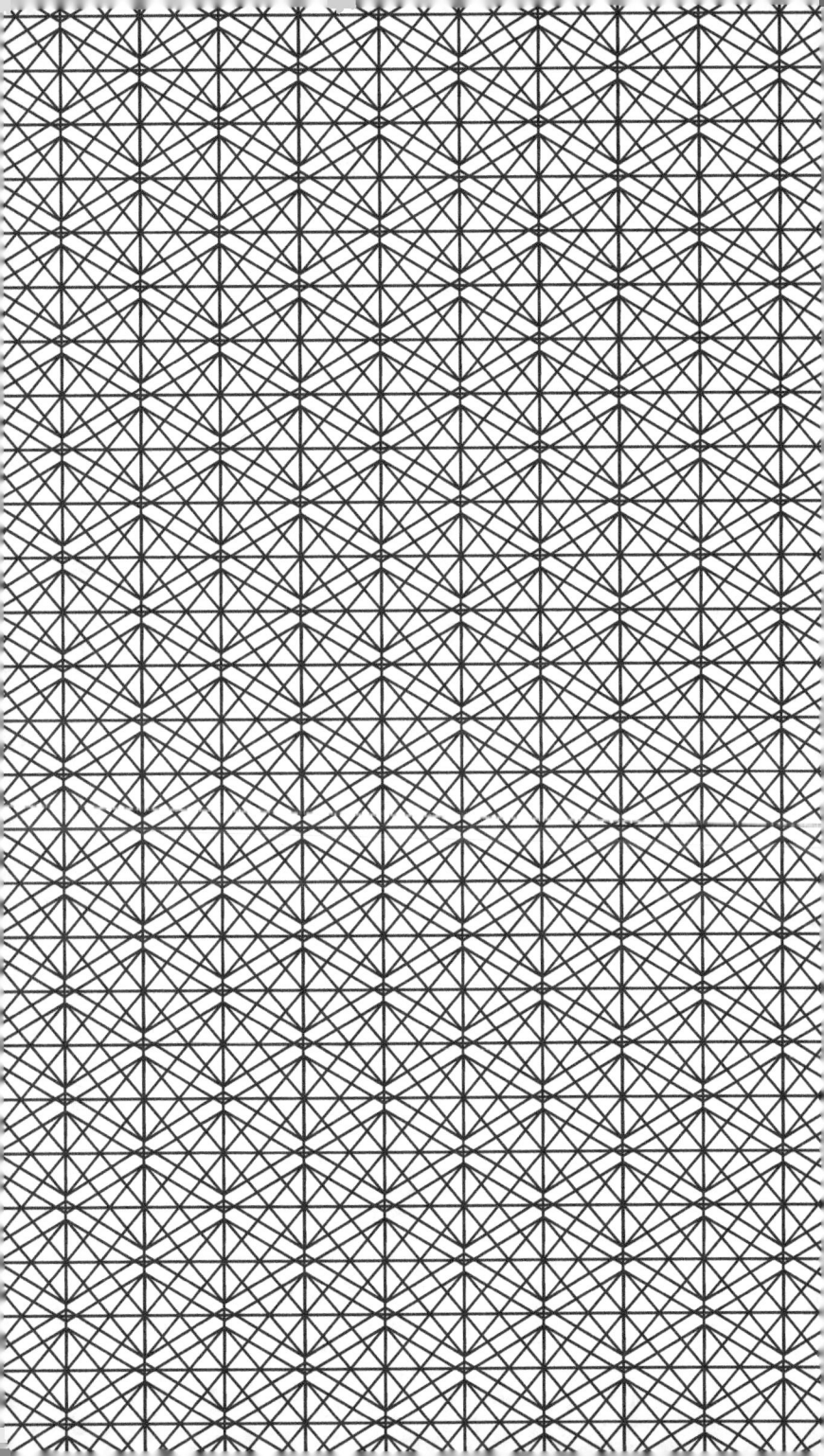

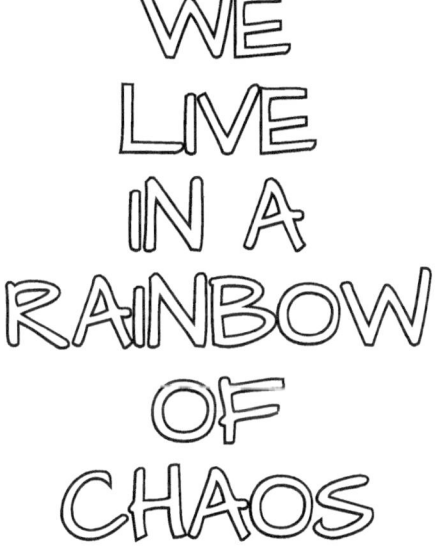

WE
LIVE
IN A
RAINBOW
OF
CHAOS

PAUL CEZANNE

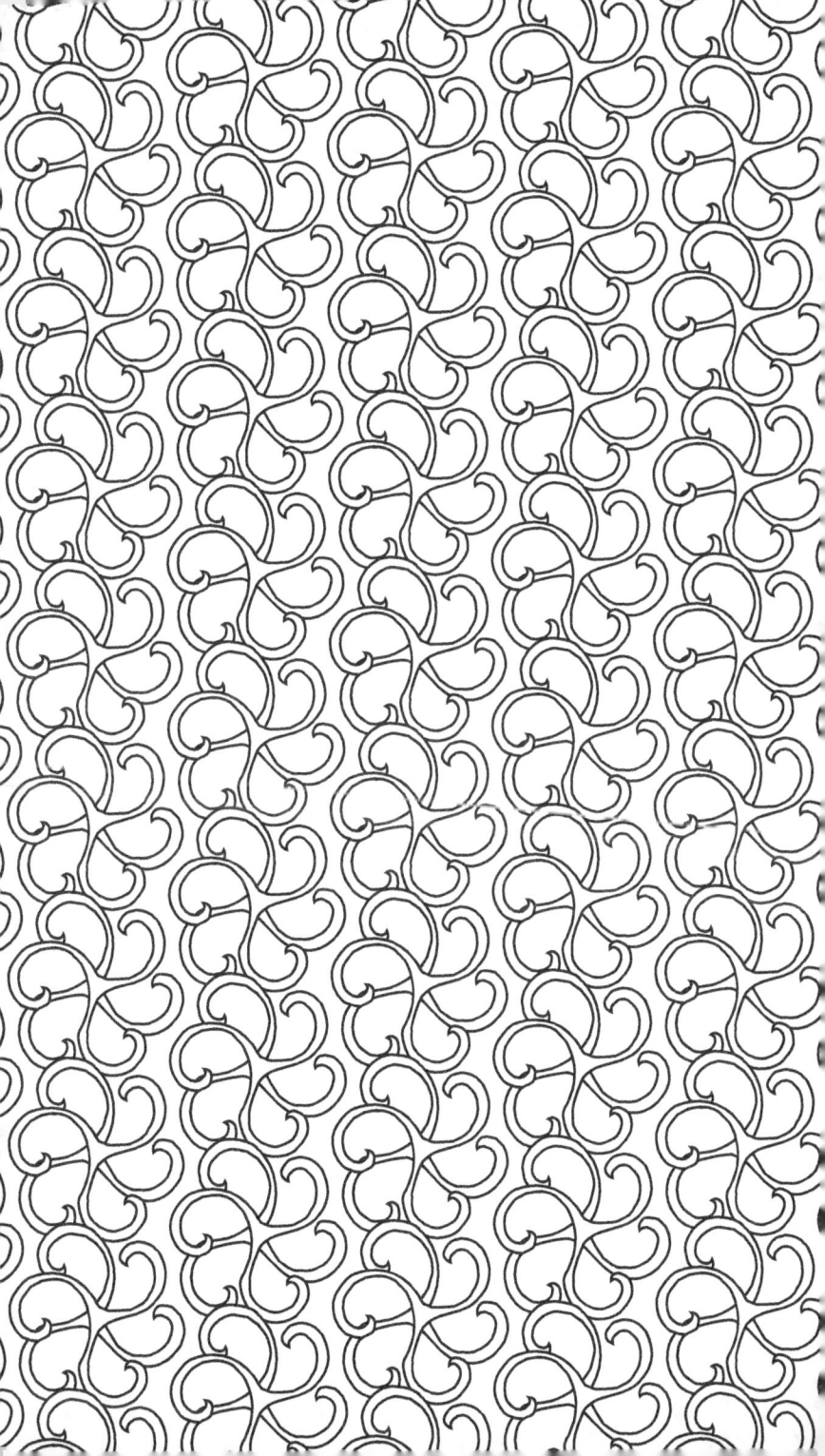

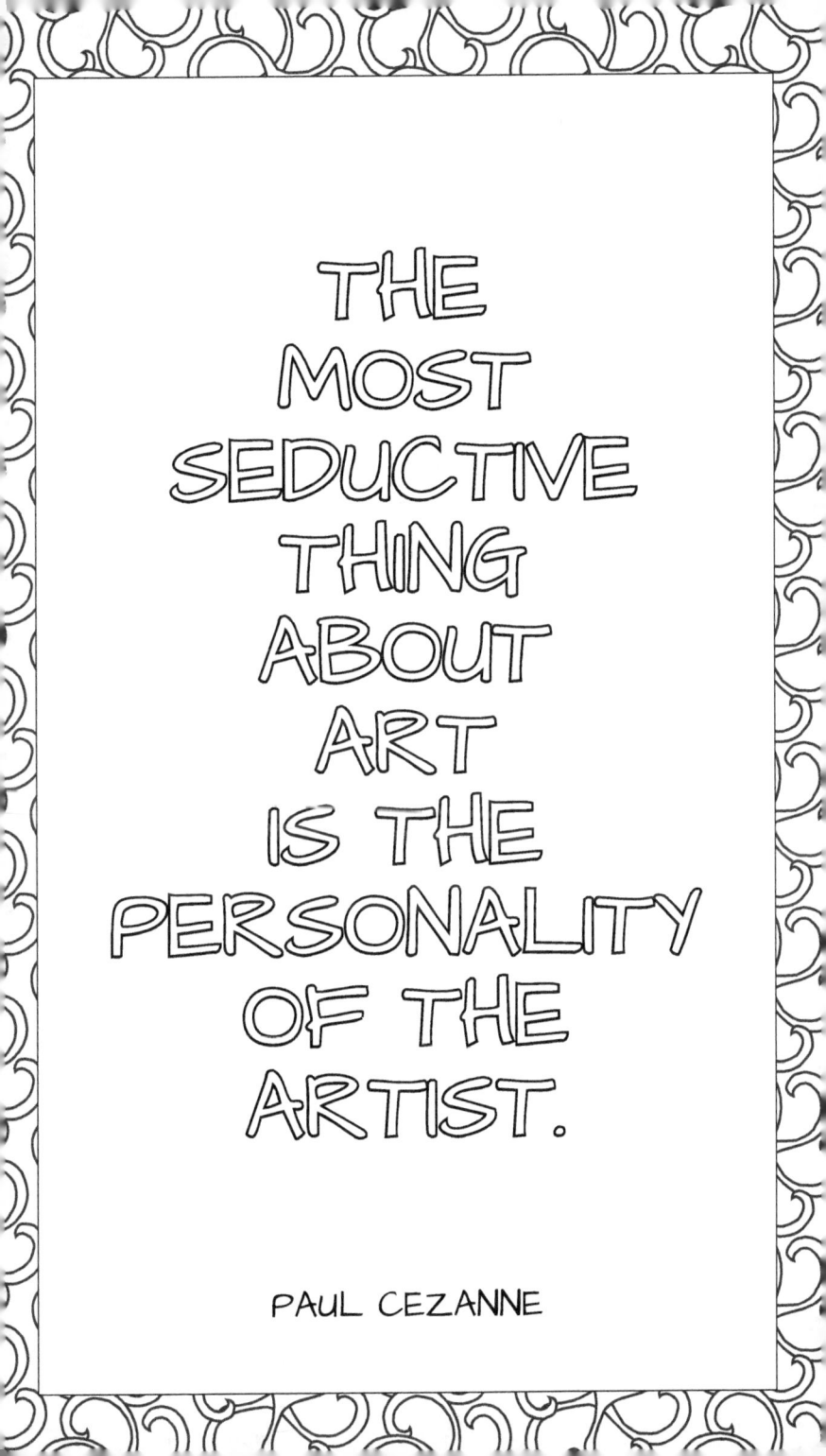

THE
MOST
SEDUCTIVE
THING
ABOUT
ART
IS THE
PERSONALITY
OF THE
ARTIST.

PAUL CEZANNE

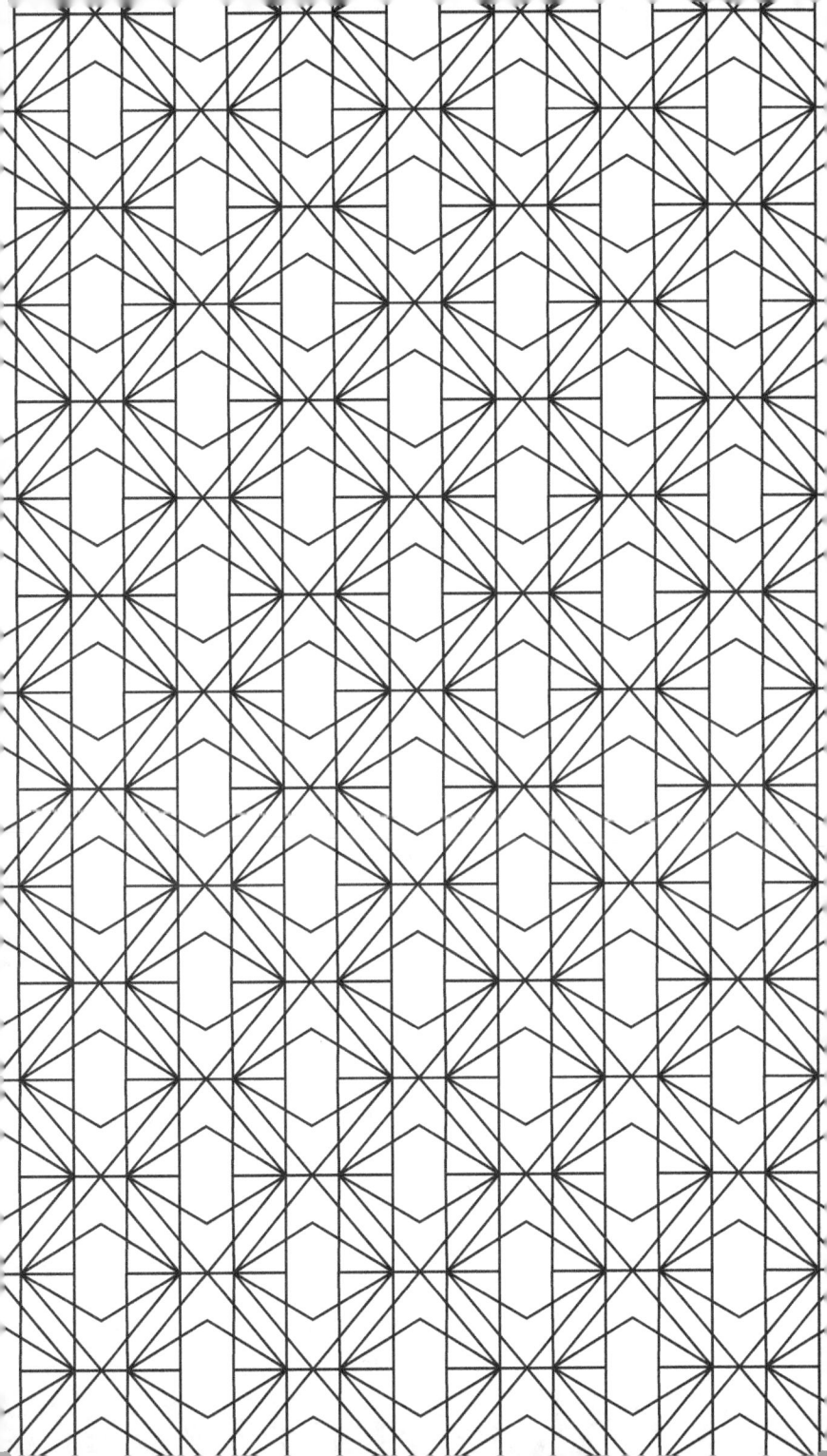

DON'T BE AN ART CRITIC, BUT PAINT

PAUL CEZANNE

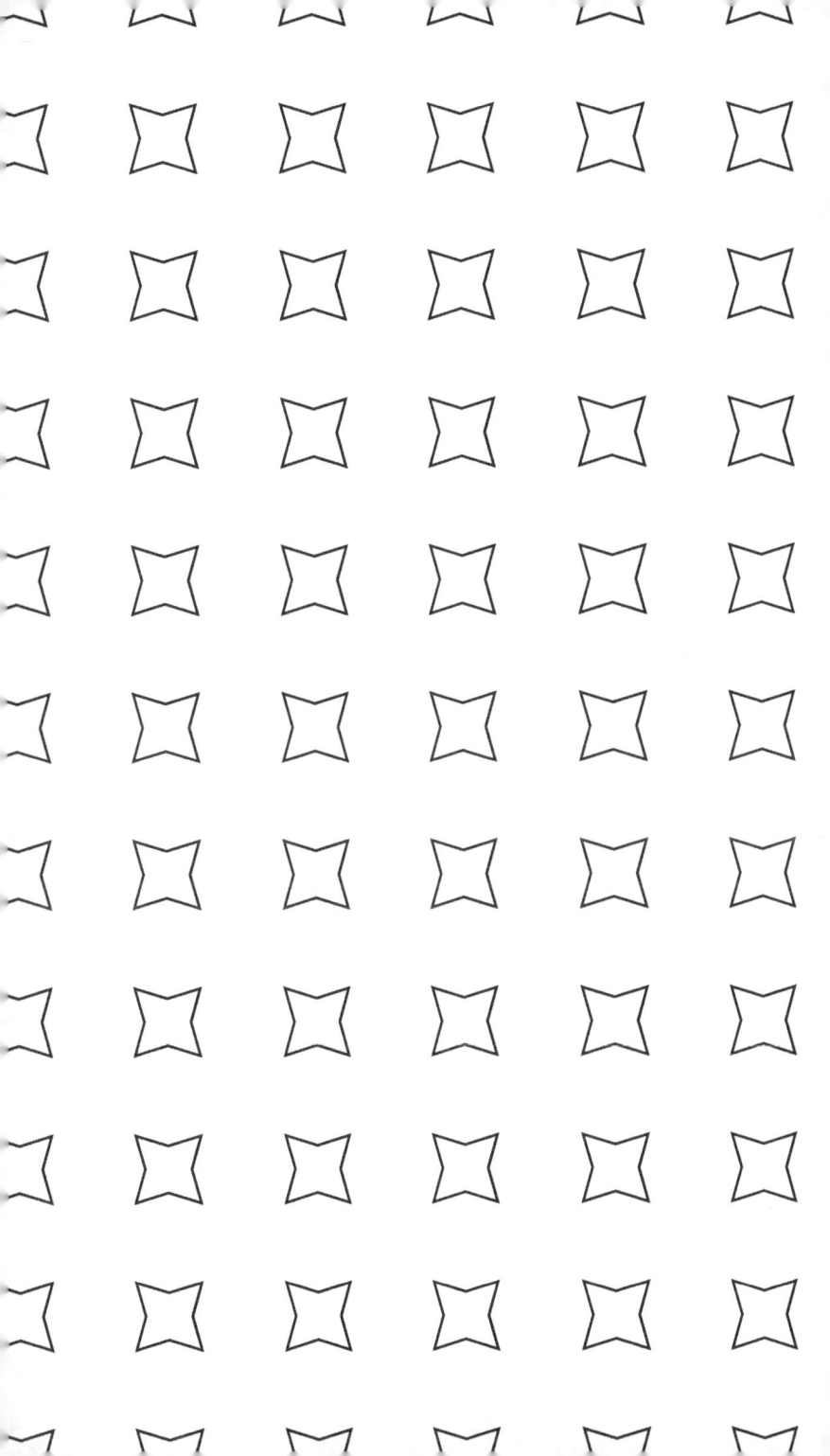

WHY COLOR?
BECAUSE
IT MAKES
THE WORLD
BIGGER,
UNVEILING
ALL THAT IS
POSSIBLE.

UNKNOWN

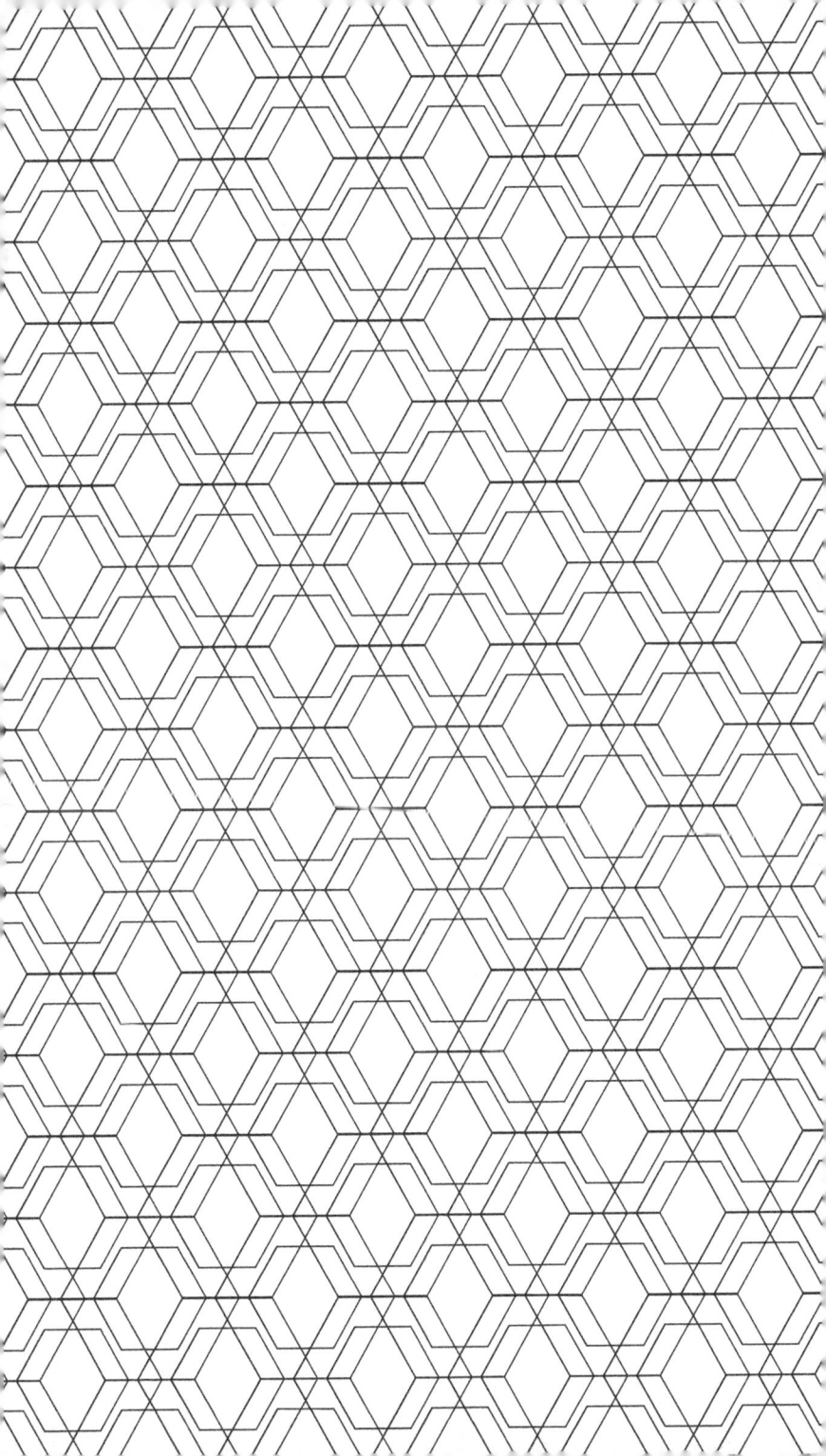

THE
PUREST
AND MOST
THOUGHTFUL
MINDS
ARE THOSE
WHICH
LOVE COLOR
THE MOST.

JOHN RUSKIN

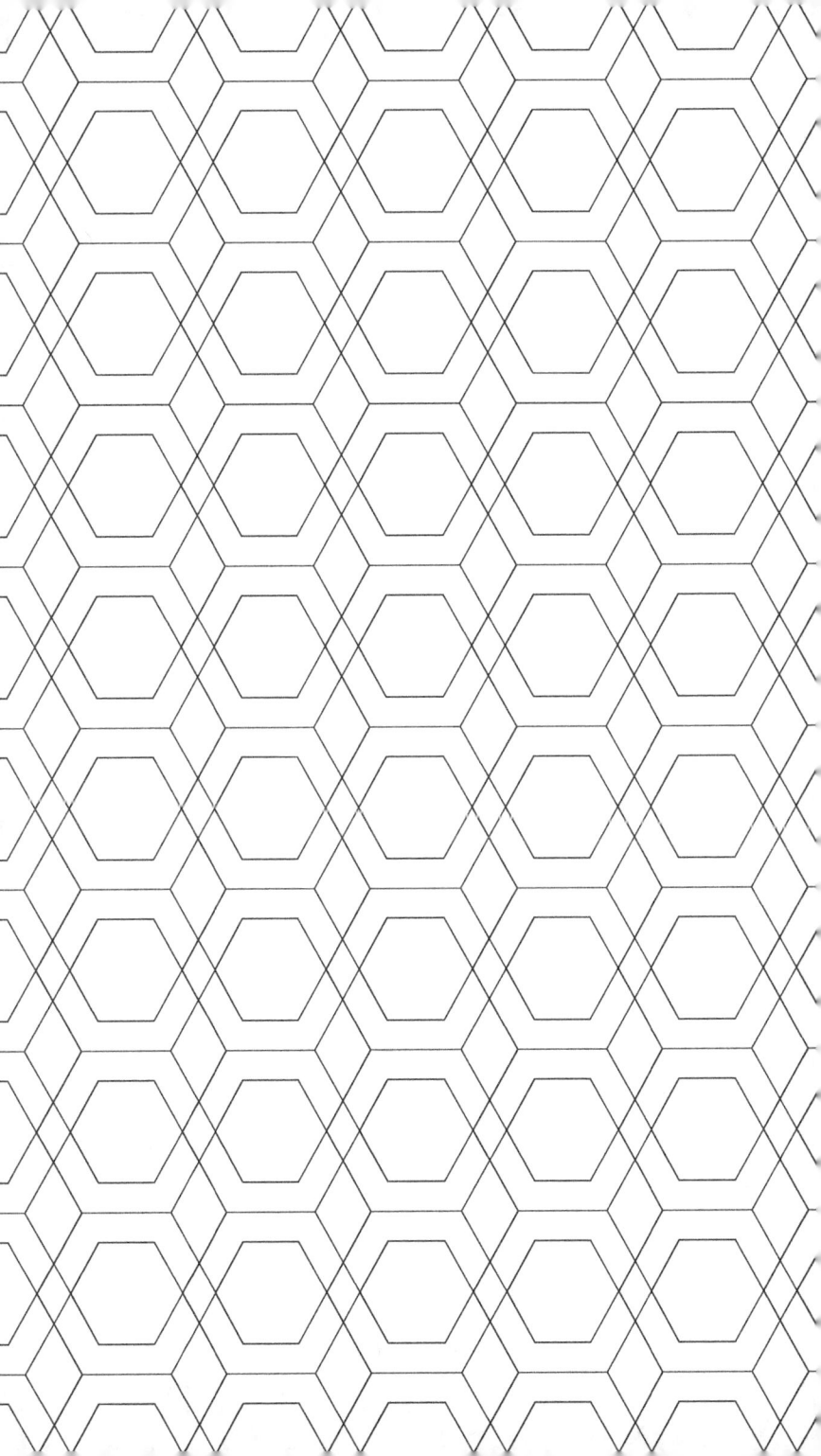

AS THE
SUN
COLORS
FLOWERS
SO DOES
ART
COLORS
LIFE.

JOHN LUBBOCK

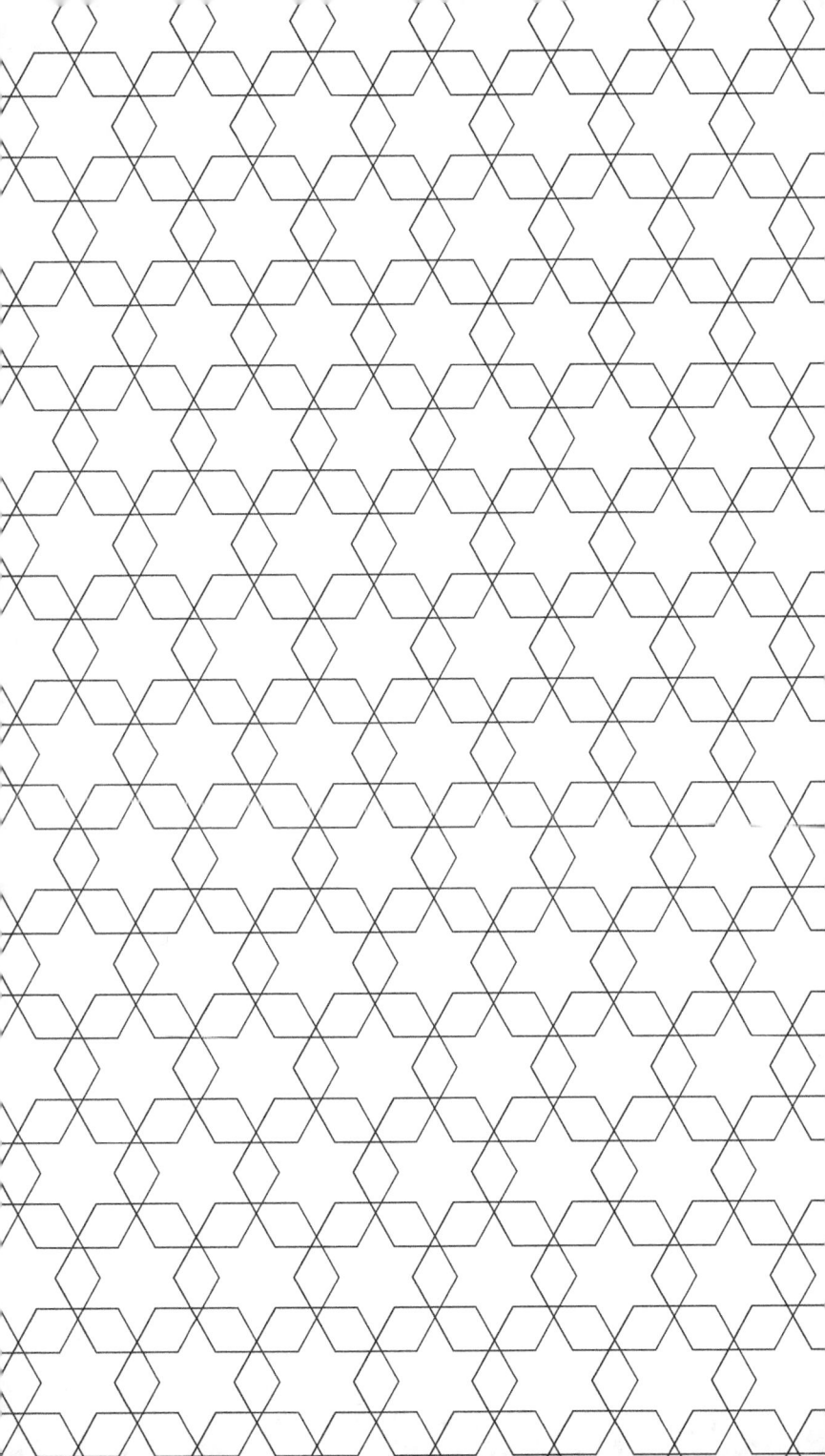

SEE WHO
WISHES TO
BECOME A
MASTER OF
COLOR MUST
SEE, FEEL,
EXPERIENCE
EACH INDIVIDUAL
COLOR IN
ITS ENDLESS
COMBINATIONS
WITH ALL
OTHER COLORS.

JOHANNES ITTEN

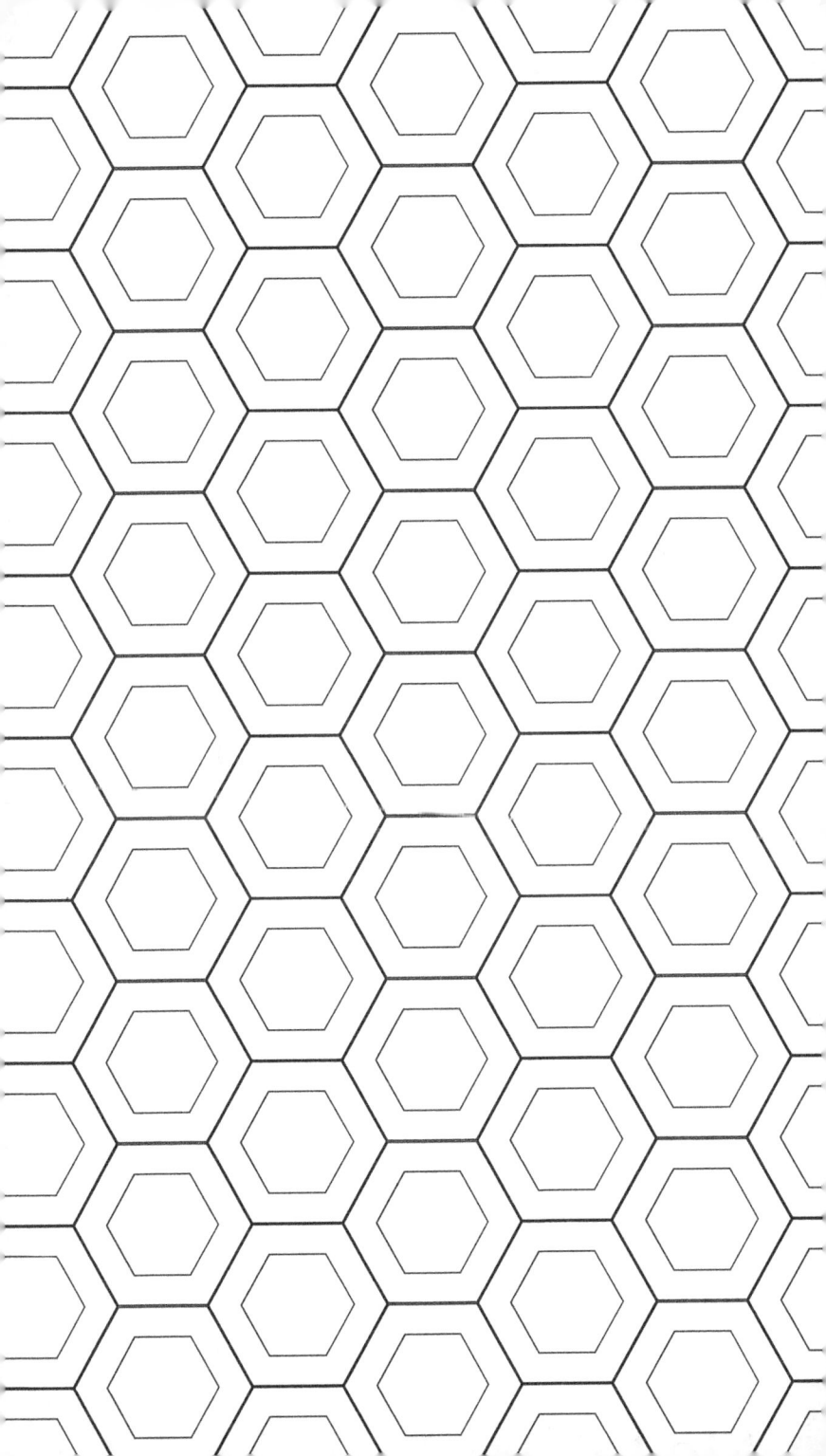

I TRY TO
APPLY
COLORS LIKE
WORDS THAT
SHAPE POEMS
LIKE NOTES
THAT SHAPE
MUSIC.

JOAN MIRO

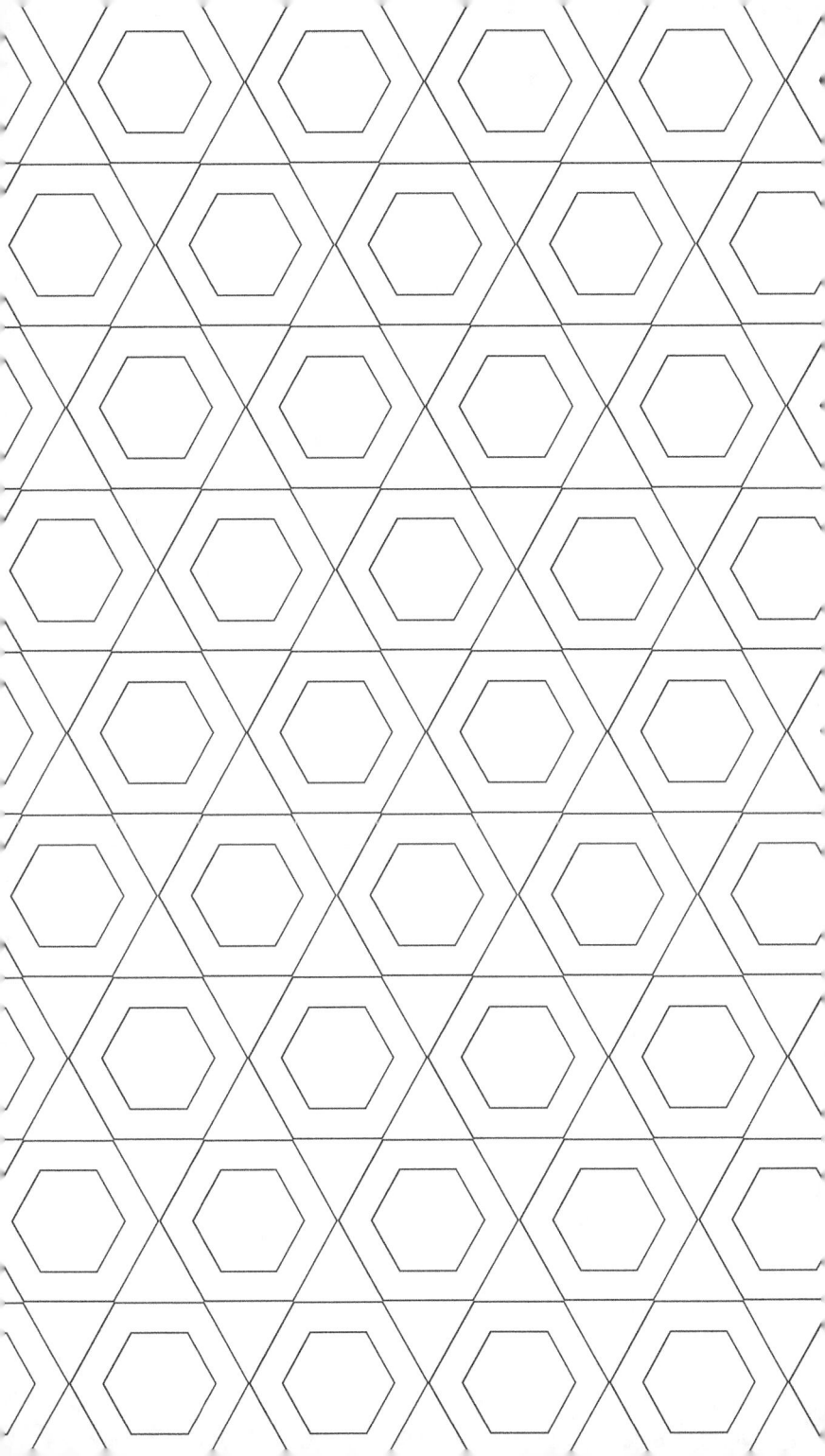

THIS MAY SOUND A BIT SIMPLE BUT THE RAINBOW WAS MY TEACHING SOURCE ABOUT MIXING COLORS.

JIM PESCOTT

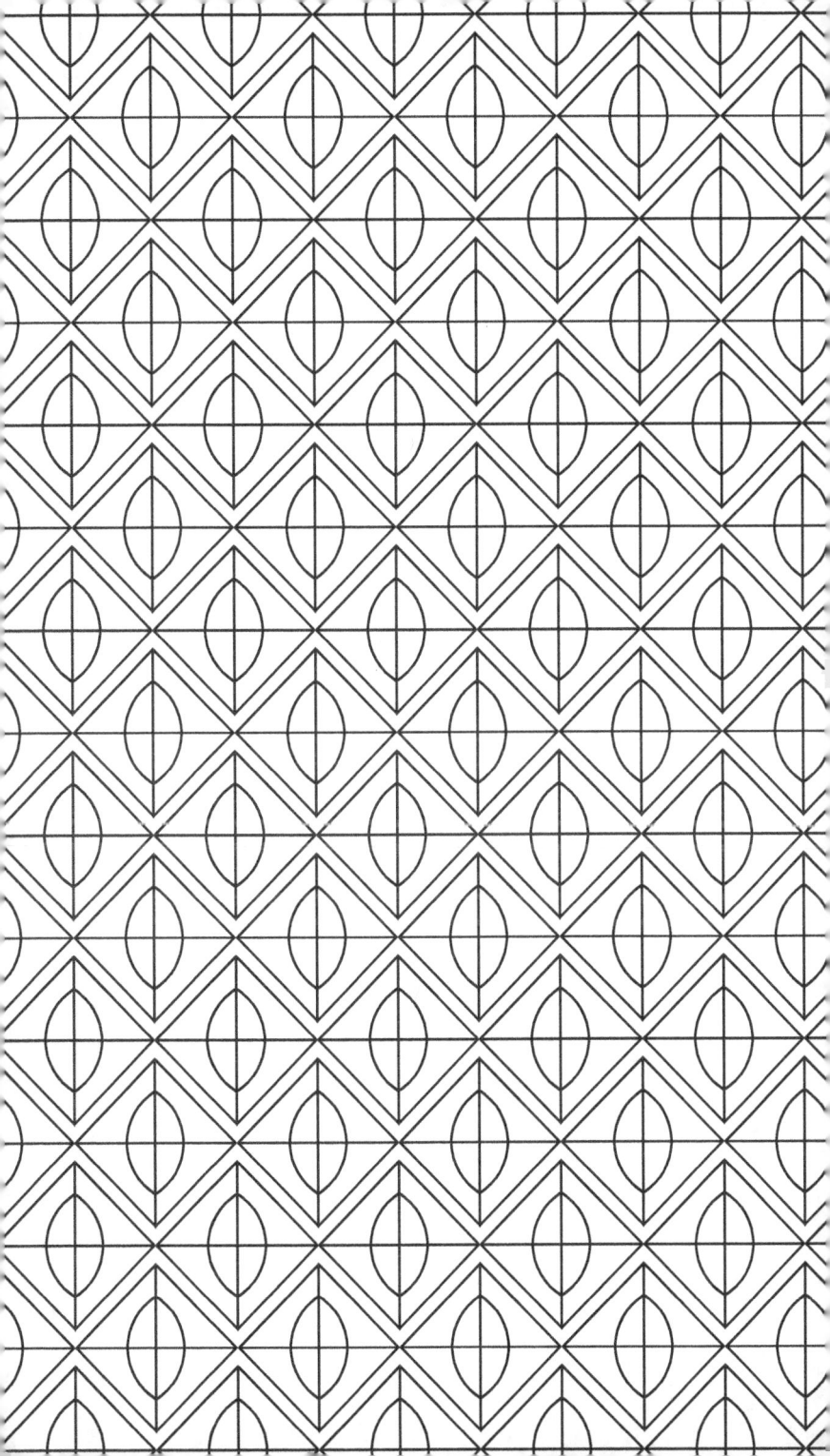

THERE IS AN
UNDENIABLE
VIRTUE TO A
TRUE BLACK
ALLOWING THE
BRAIN TO BE
MESMERIZED
AND PULLING
THE PUPILS
DEEP INTO THAT
UNFOUND BUT
SENSED
ABYSS.

JAMIE LAVIN

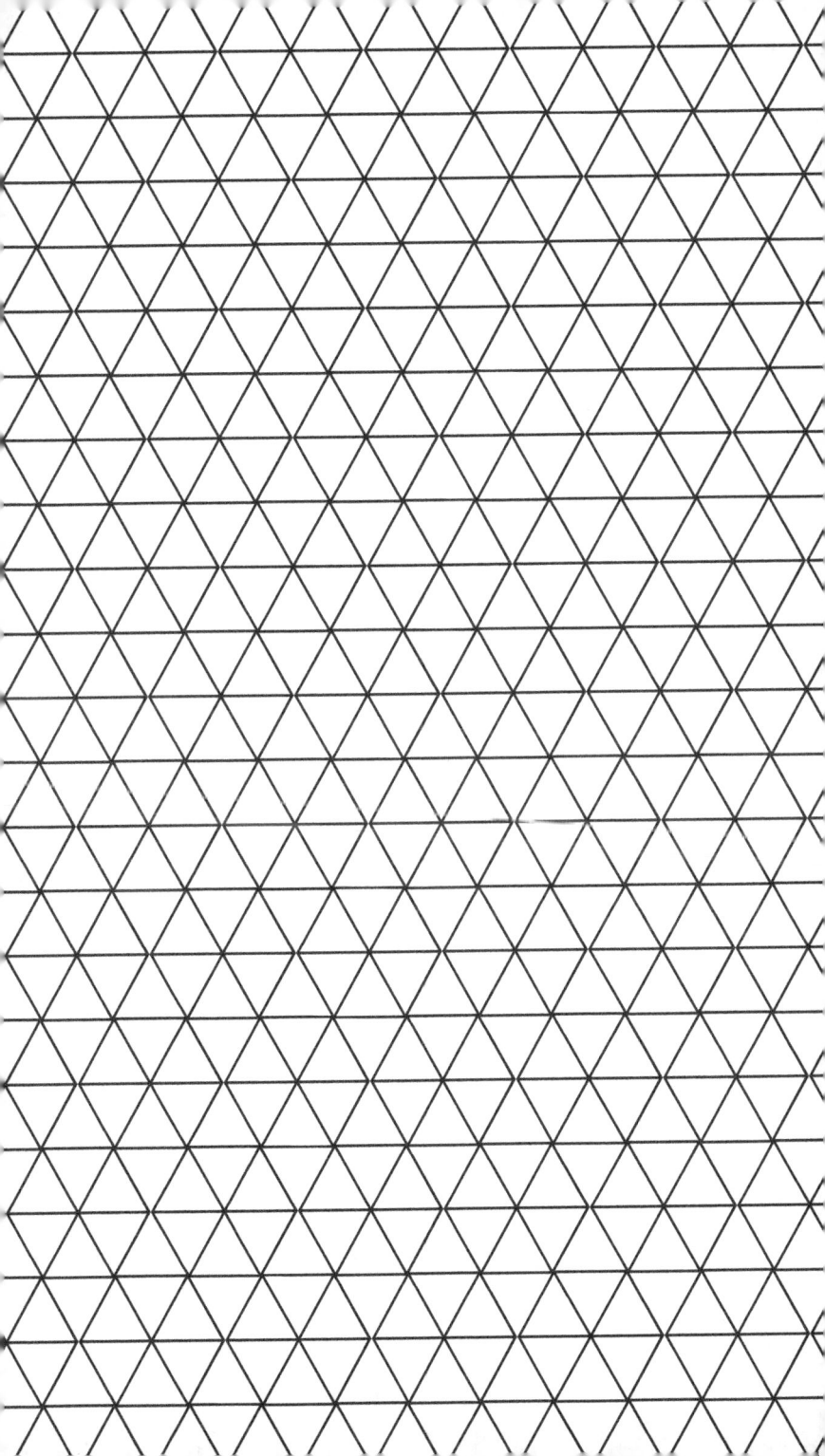

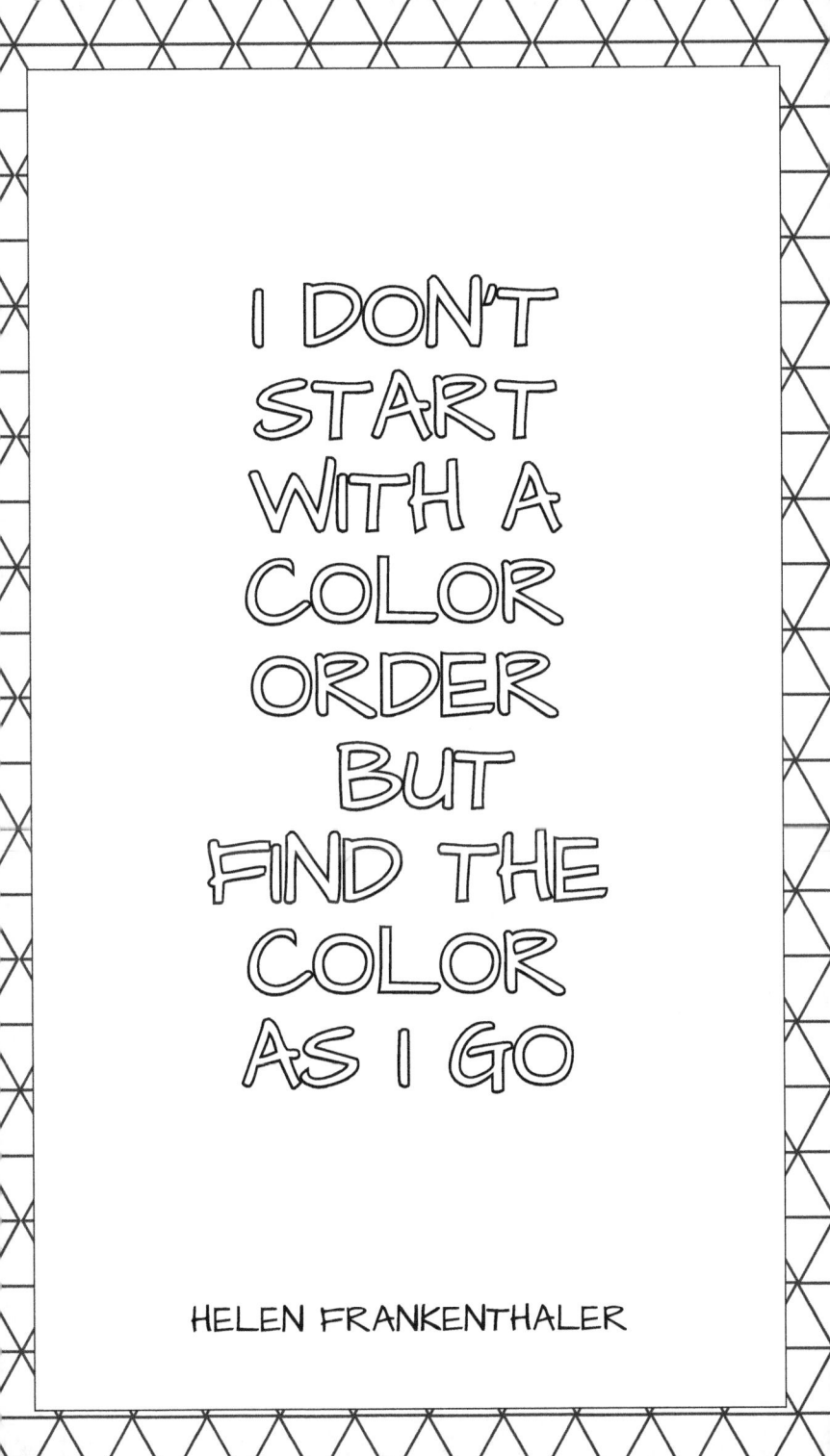

I DON'T START WITH A COLOR ORDER BUT FIND THE COLOR AS I GO

HELEN FRANKENTHALER

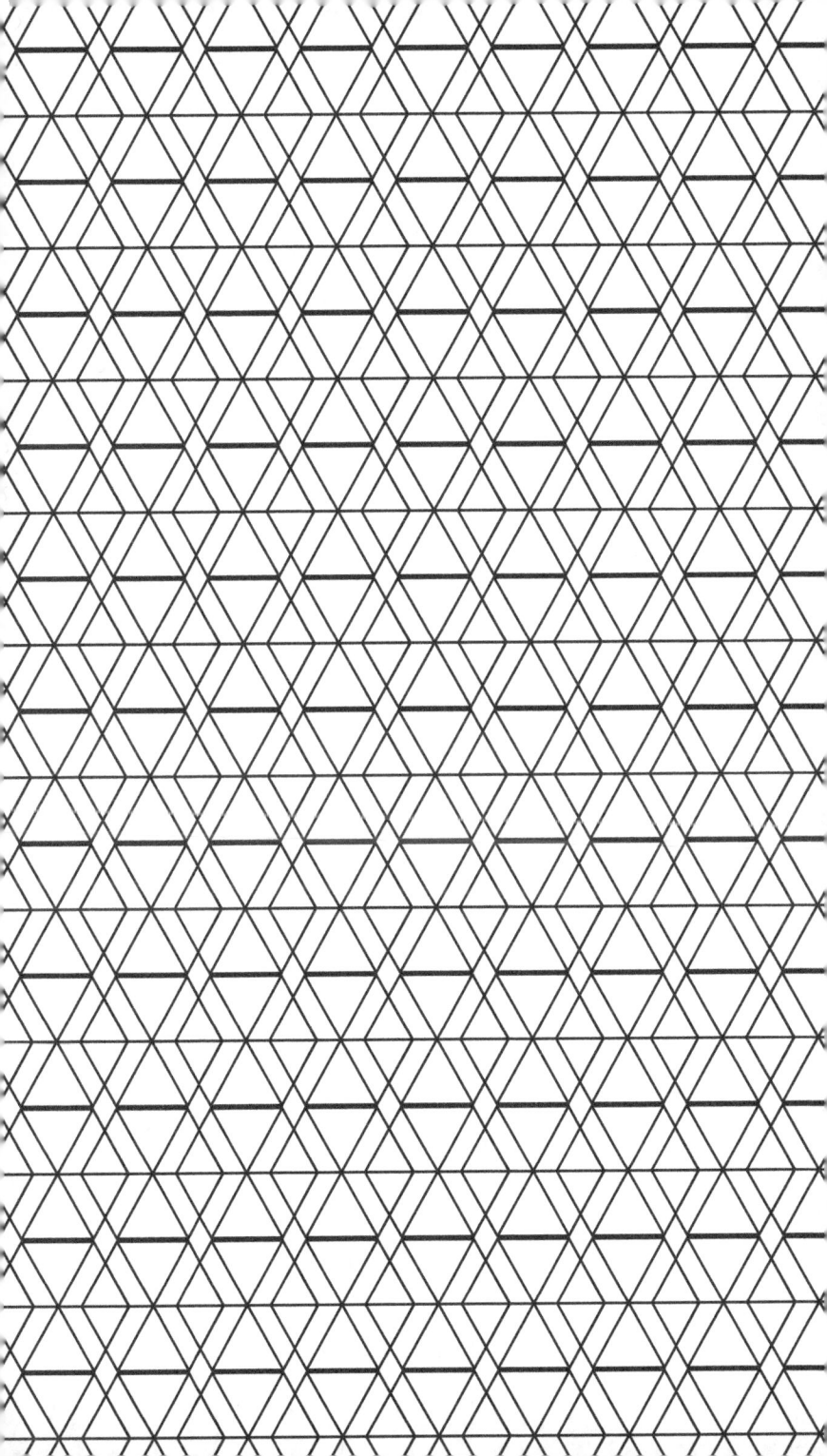

MAUVE ?
MAUVE
IS JUST
PINK
TRYING
TO BE
PURPLE !

JAMES ABBOT MCNEIL WHISTLER

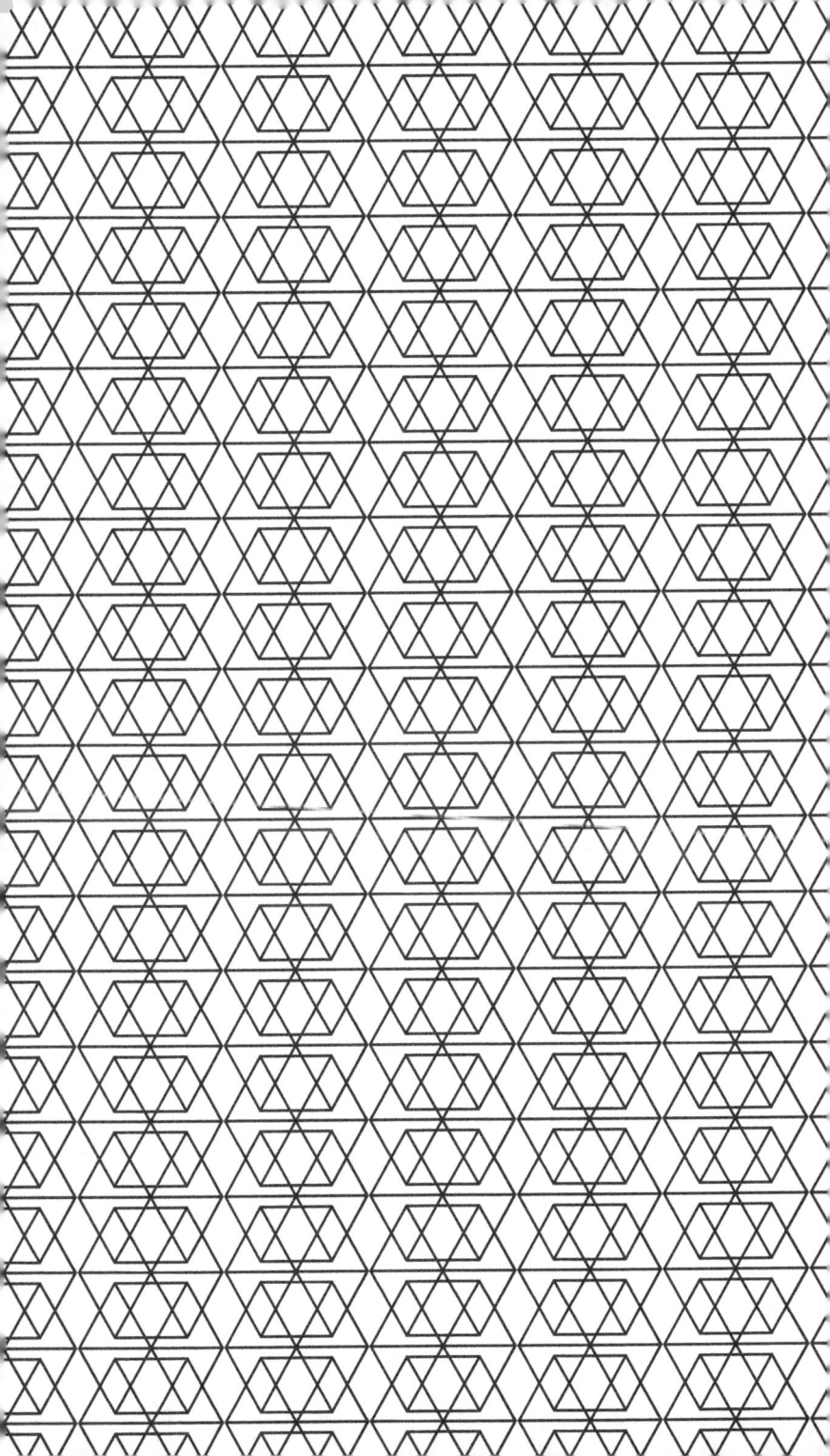

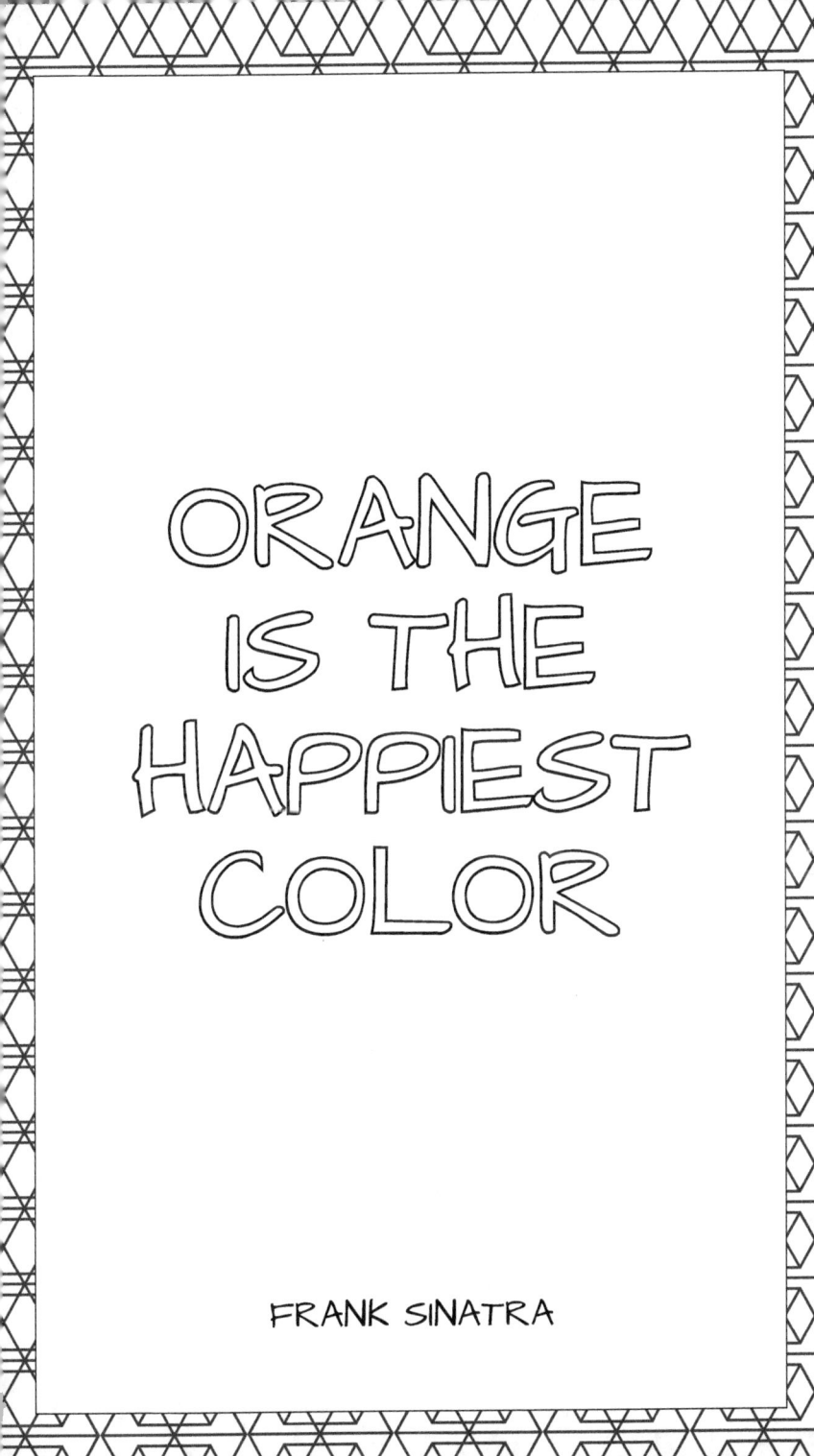

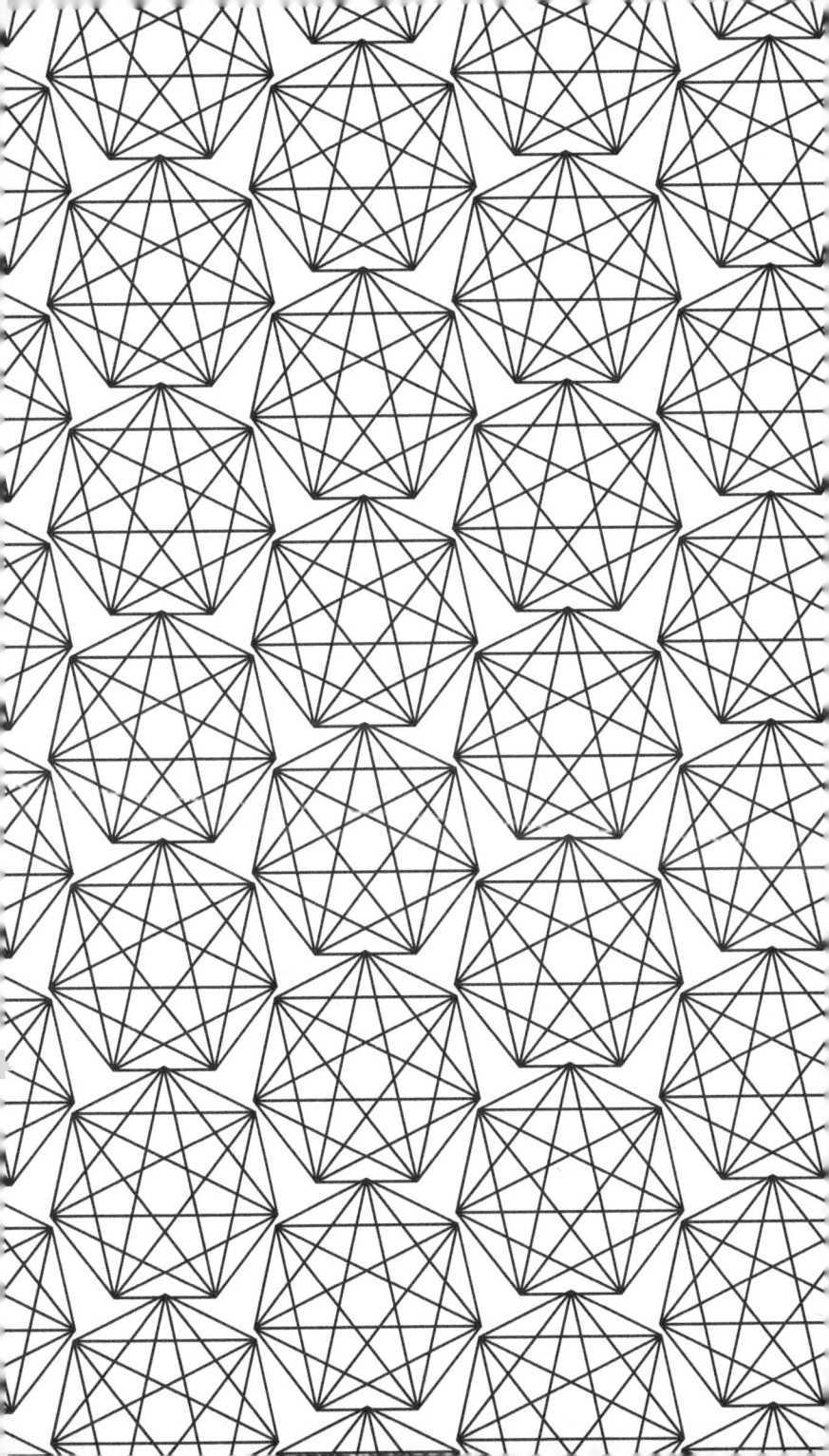

COLOR MUST FIT TOGETHER AS PIECES IN A PUZZLE OR COG IN A WHEEL.

HANS HOFMANN

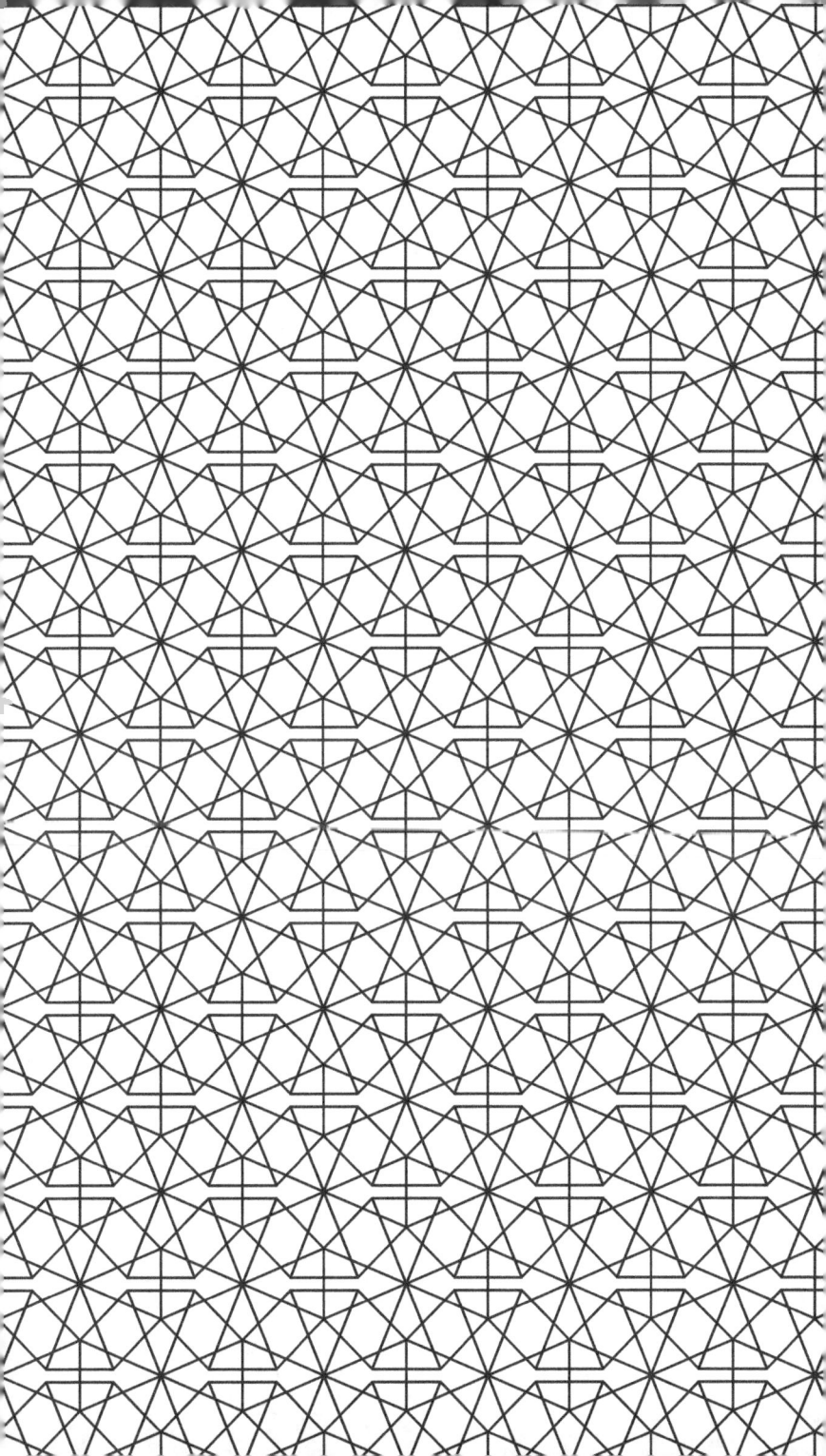

ALL COLORS AGREE IN THE DARK

FRANCIS BACON

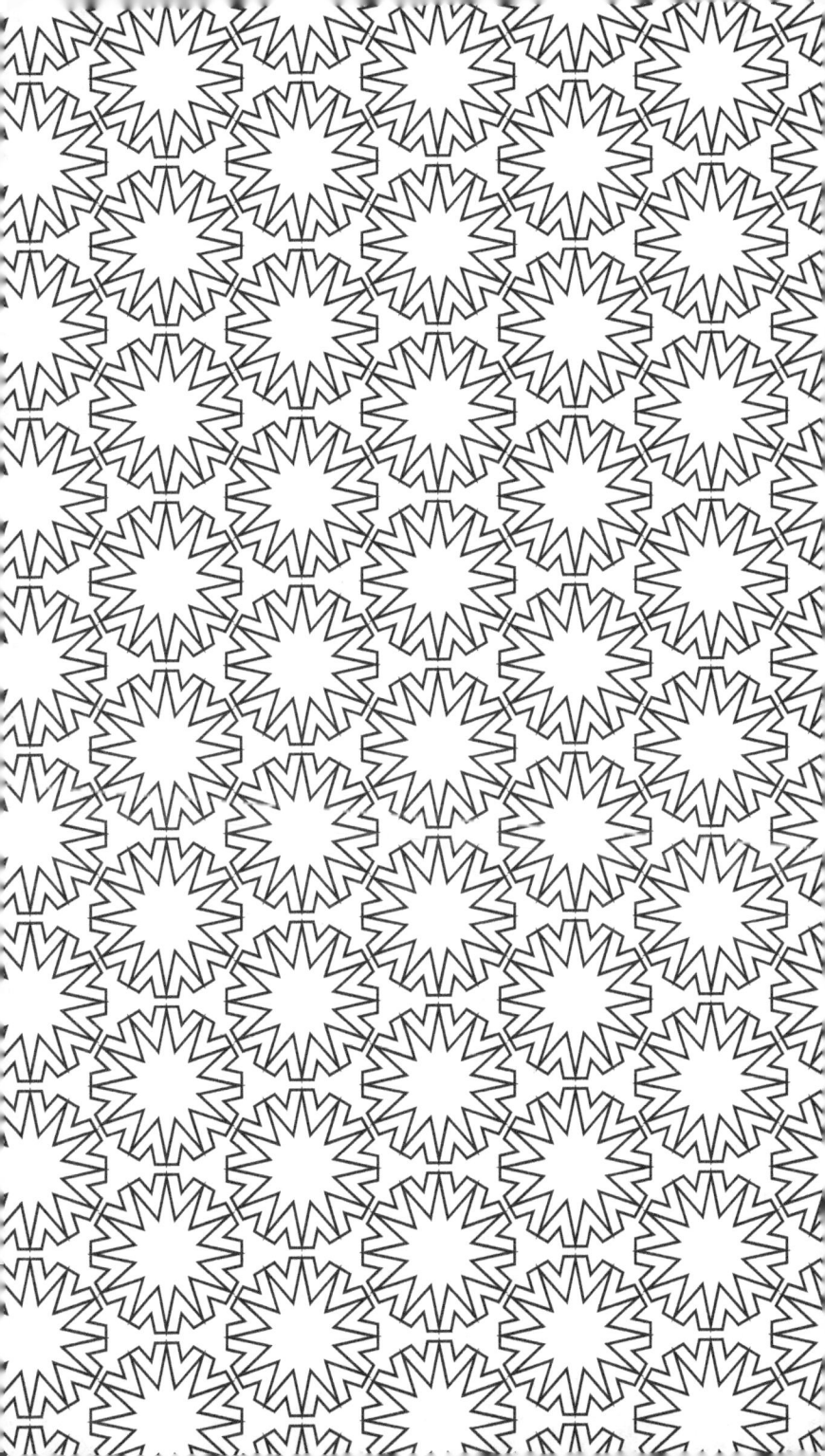

ANY
COLOR
WORKS
IF YOU PUSH
IT TO THE
EXTREME.

MASSIMO VIGNELLI

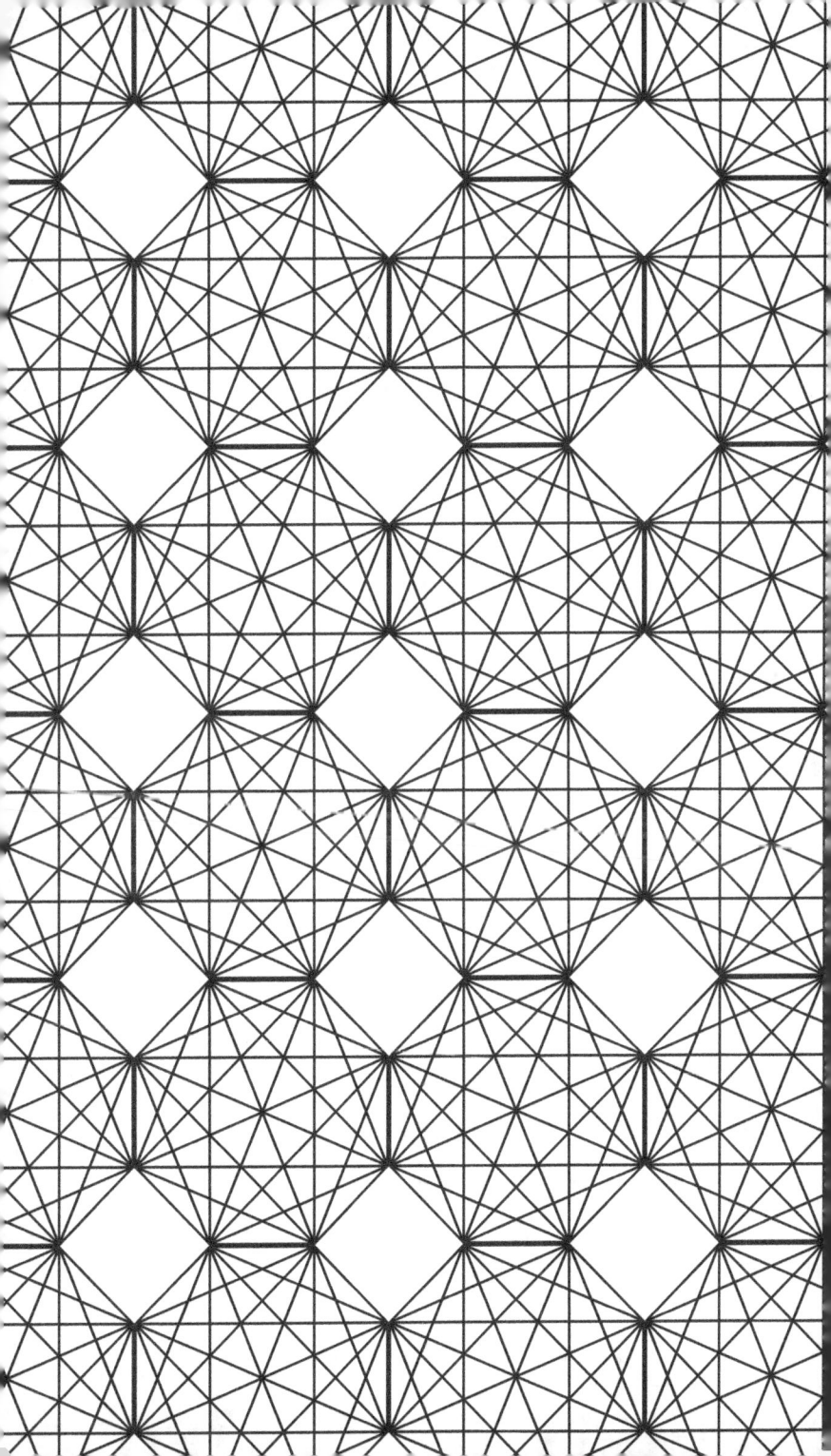

CREATIVITY
IS ALLOWING
YOURSELF
TO MAKE
MISTAKES.
ART IS
KNOWING
WHICH ONE
TO KEEP

SCOTT ADAMS

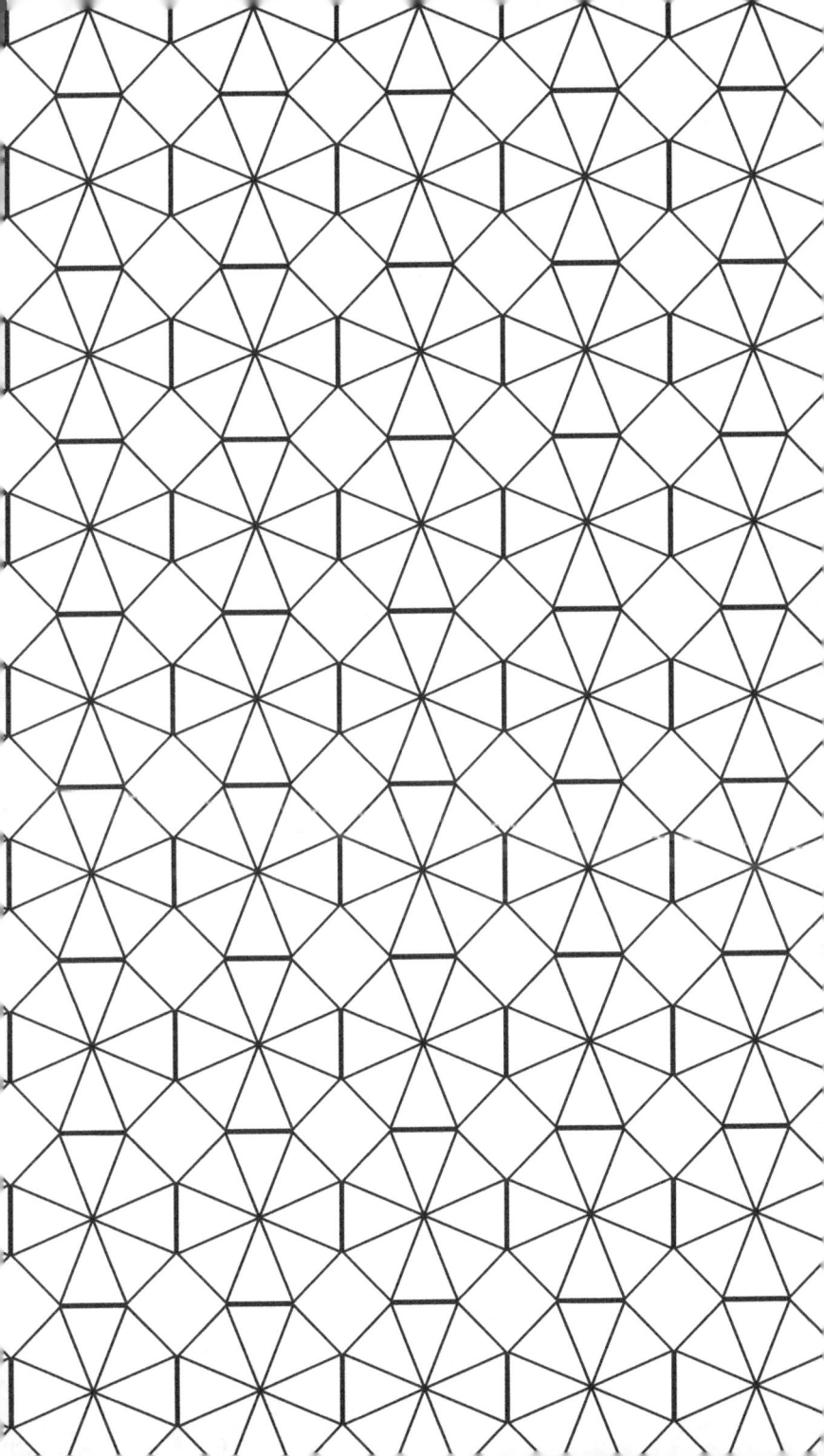

THIS
WORLD
IS BUT A
CANVAS
TO OUR
IMAGINATION

HENRY DAVID THOREAU

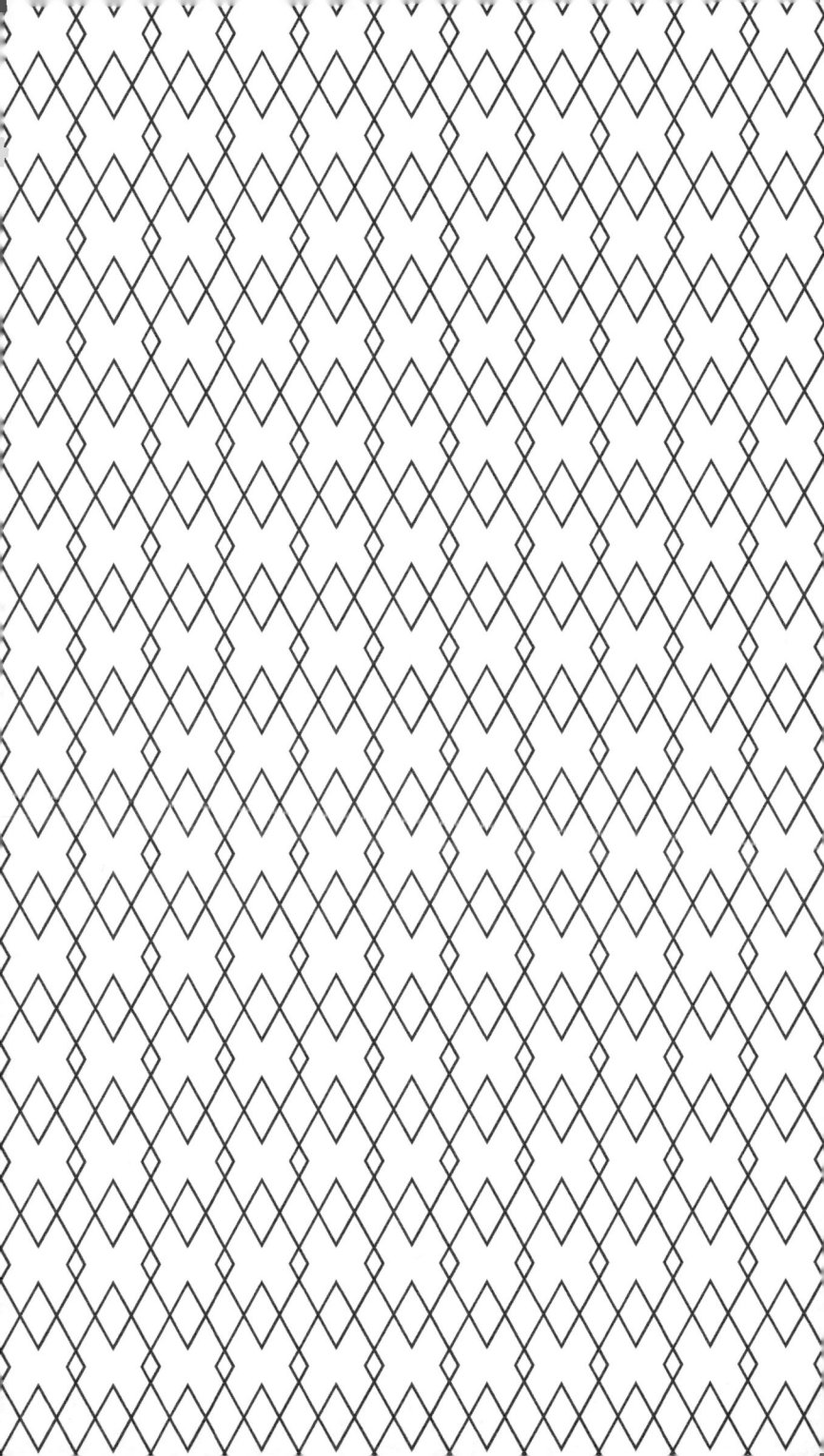

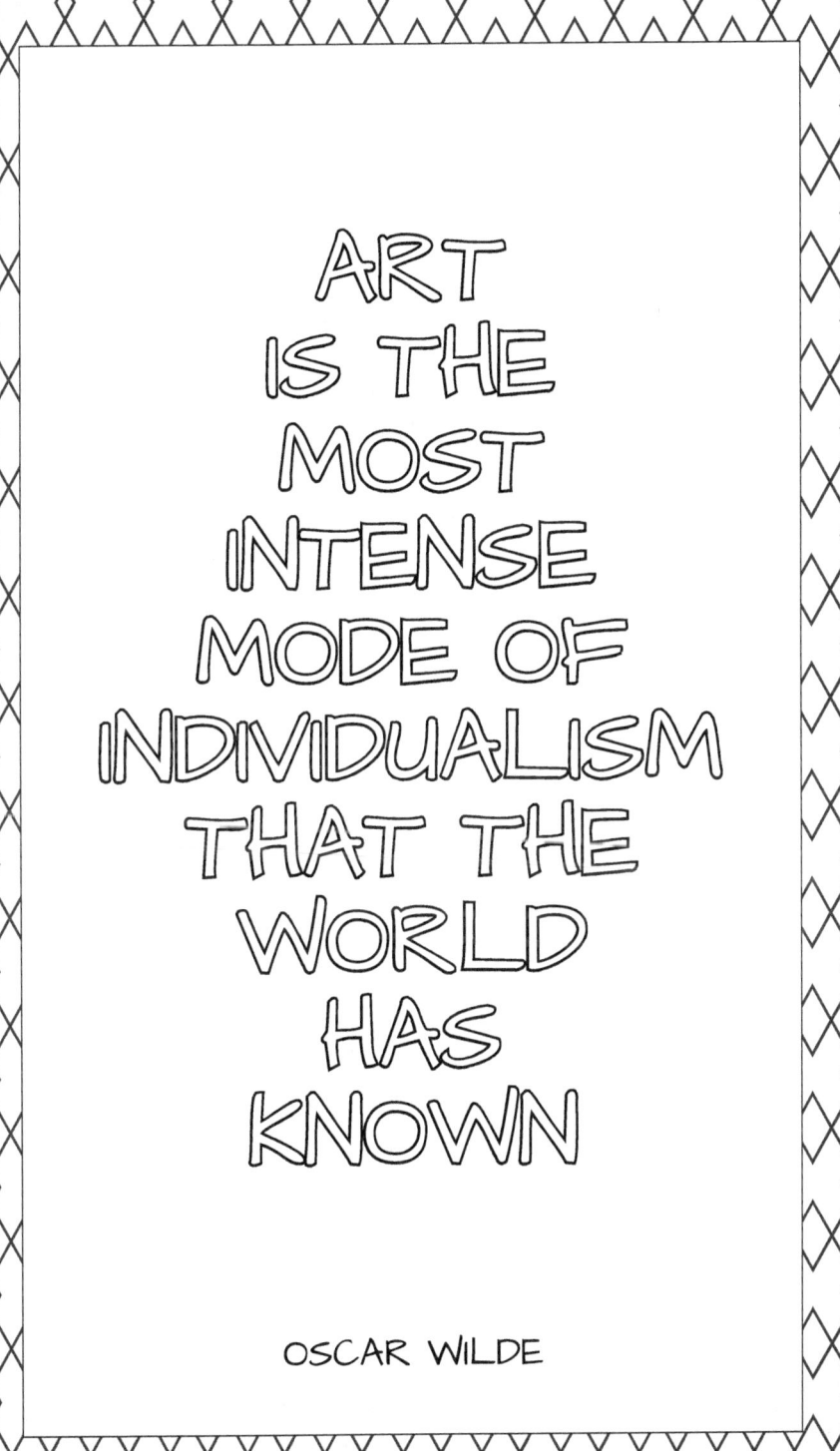

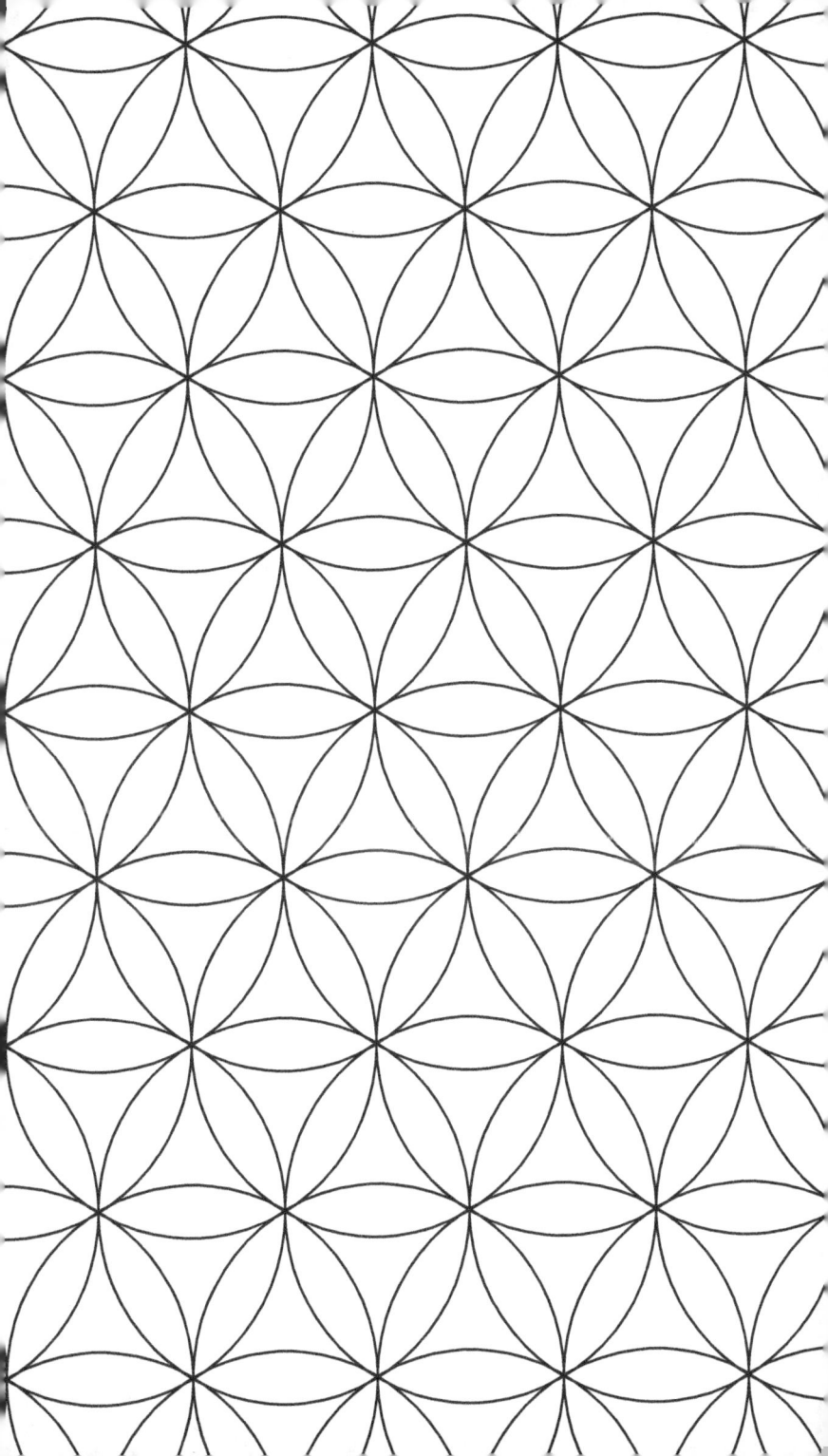

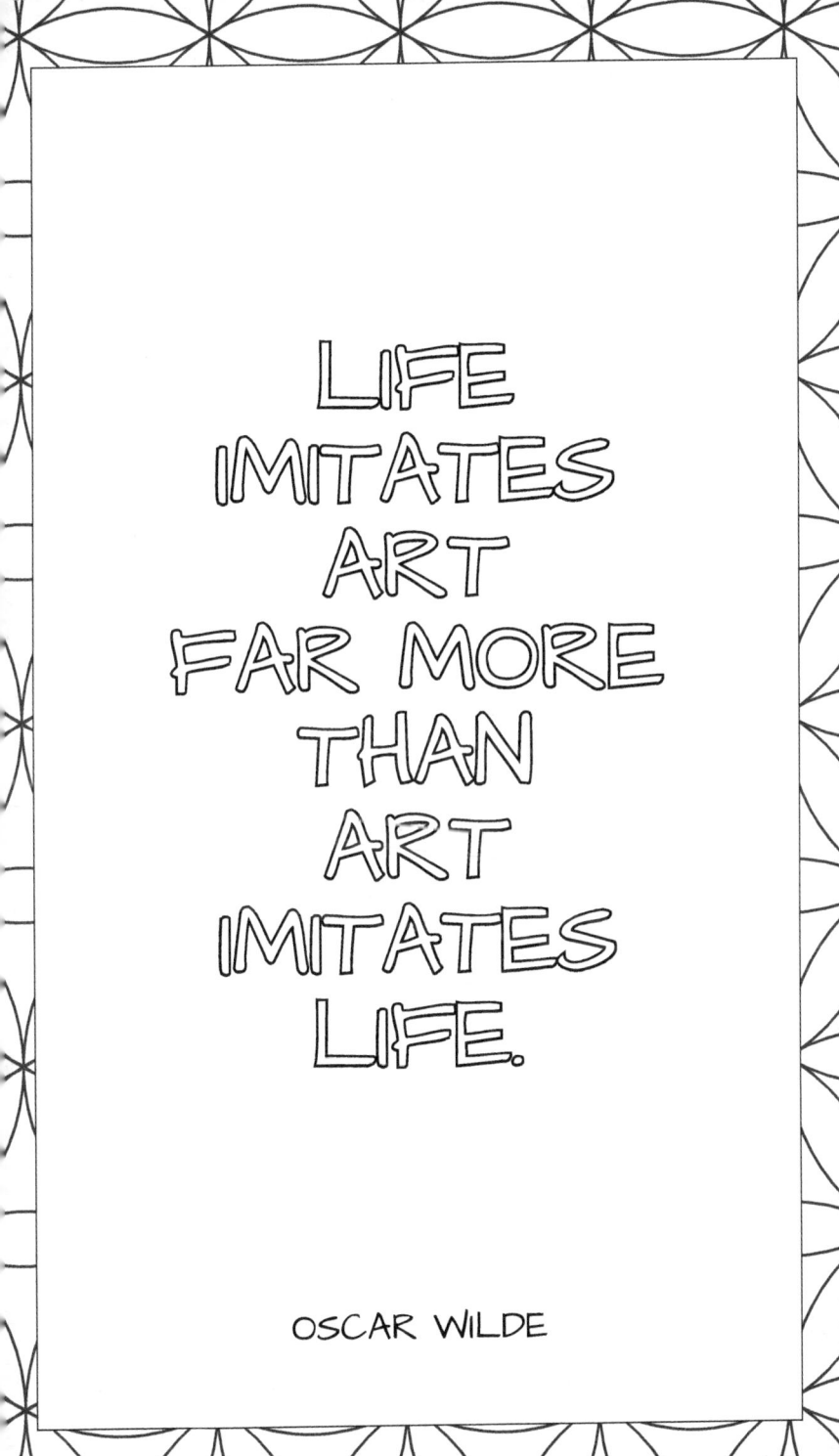

BE DRAWN
TO THE
VISUAL ART
FOR IT CAN
EXPAND YOUR
IMAGINATION.

BARBARA JANUSZKIEWICZ

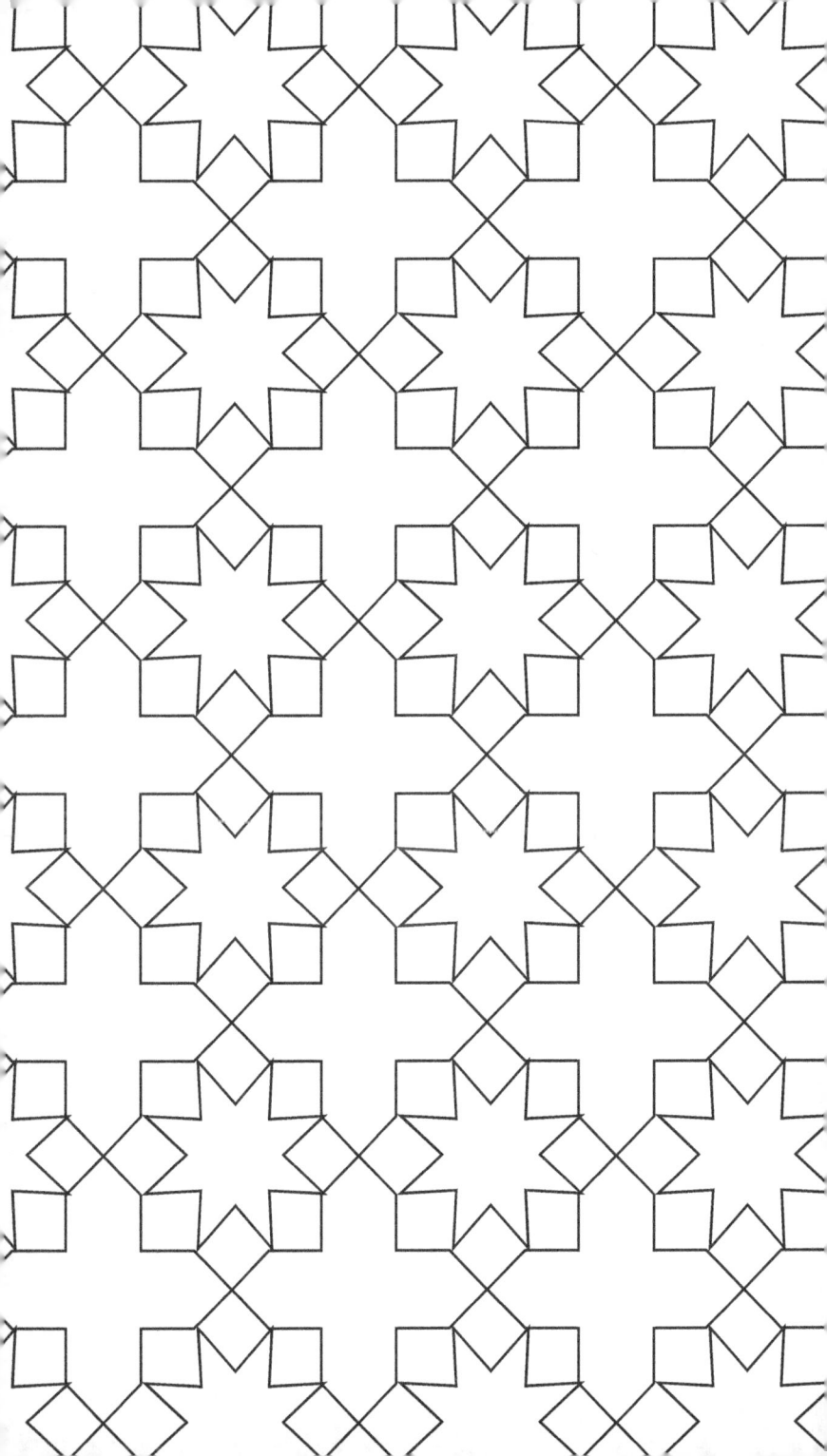

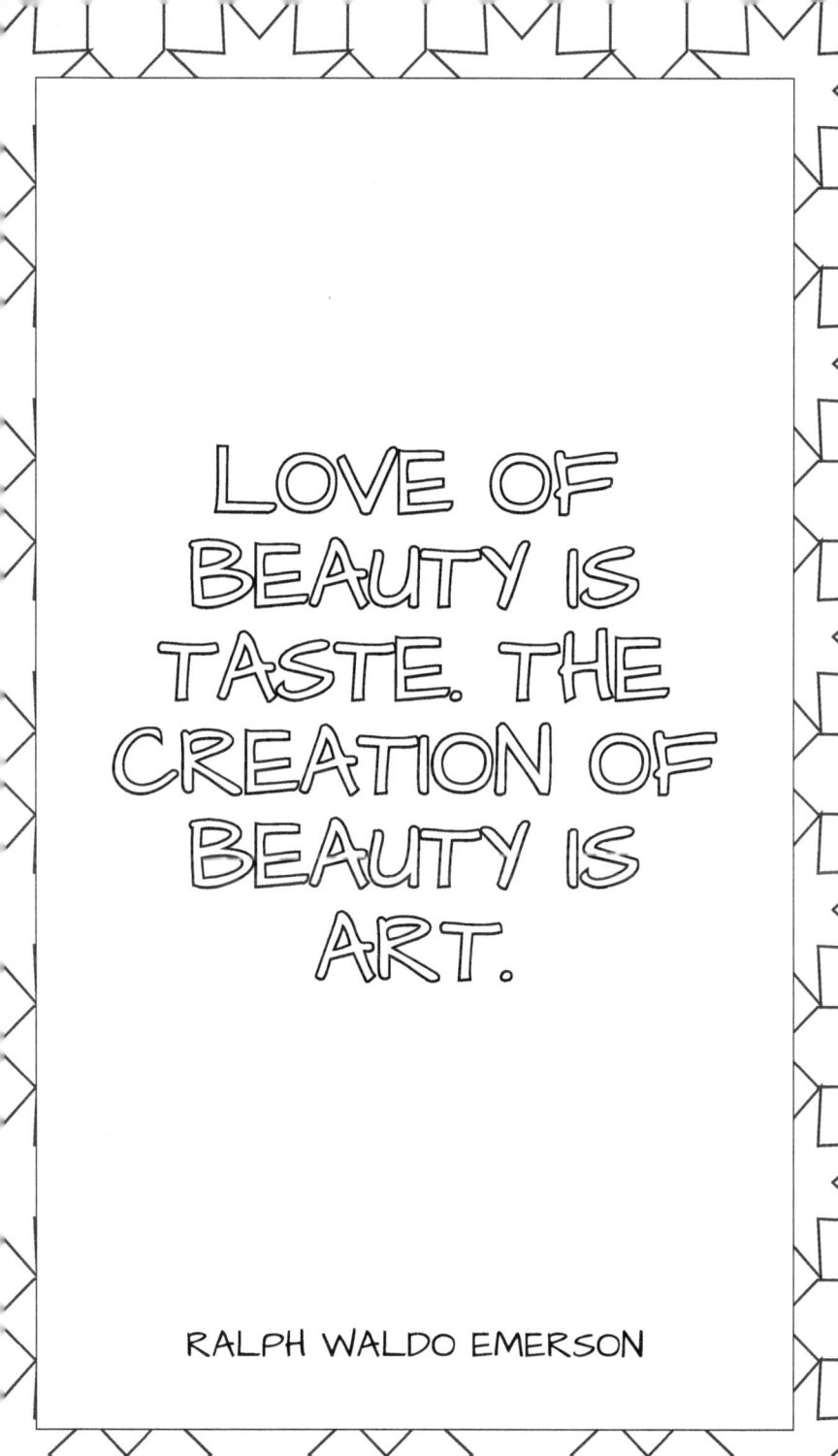

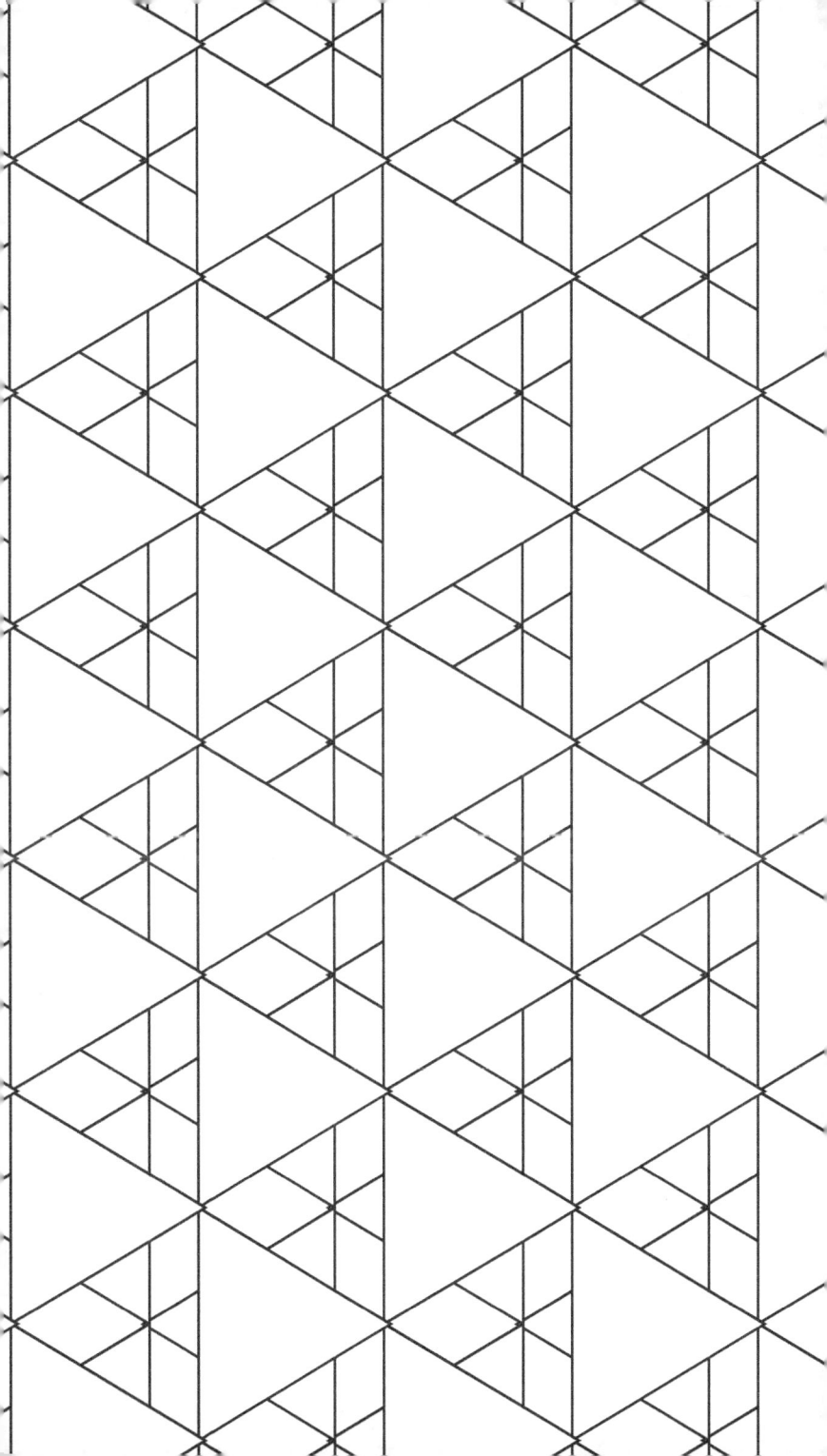

TRUE ART IS CHARACTERIZED BY AN IRRESISTIBLE URGE IN THE CREATIVE ARTIST.

ALBERT EINSTEIN

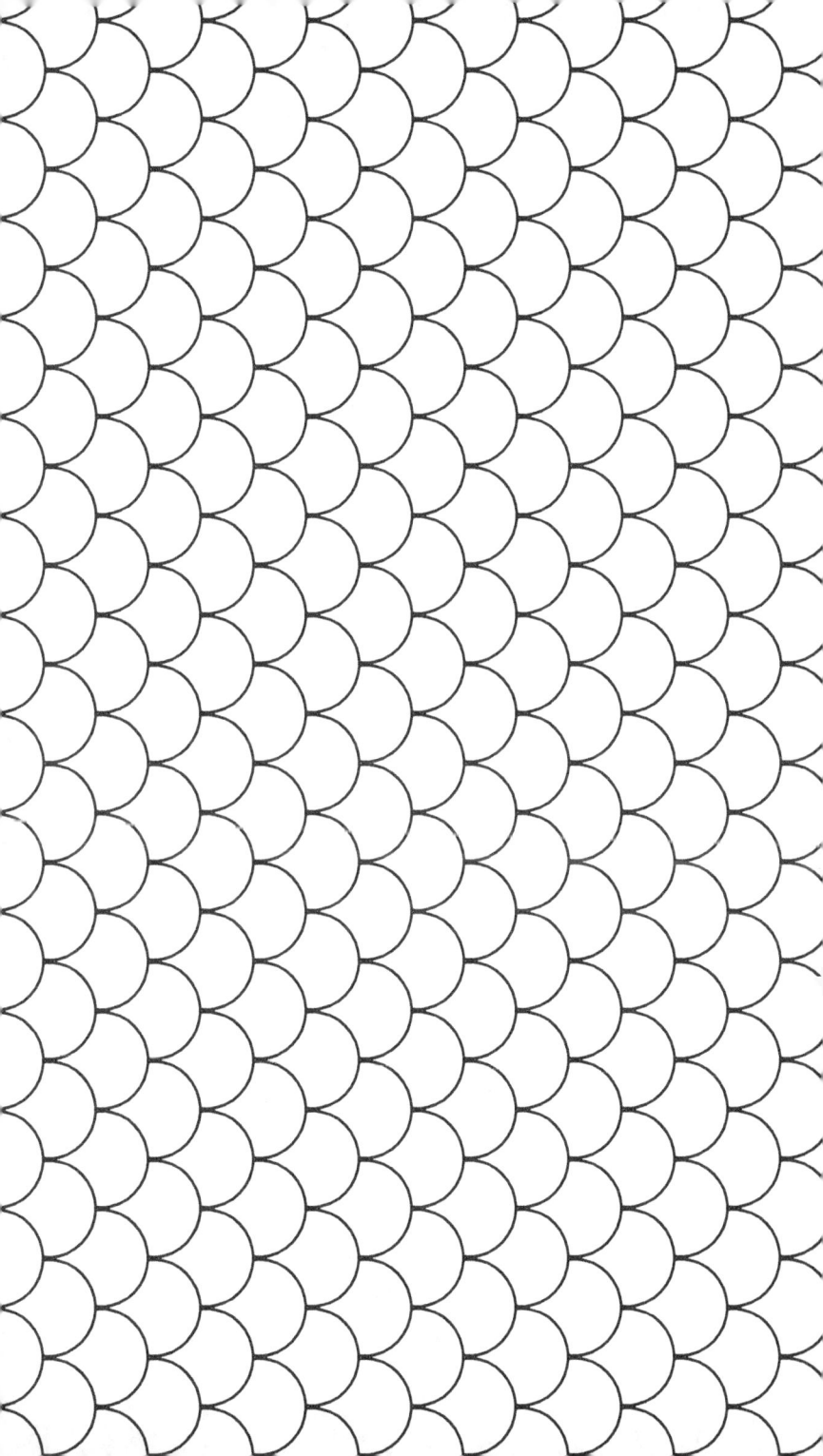

YOU CAN'T USE UP CREATIVITY. THE MORE YOU USE, THE MORE YOU HAVE.

MAYA ANGELOU

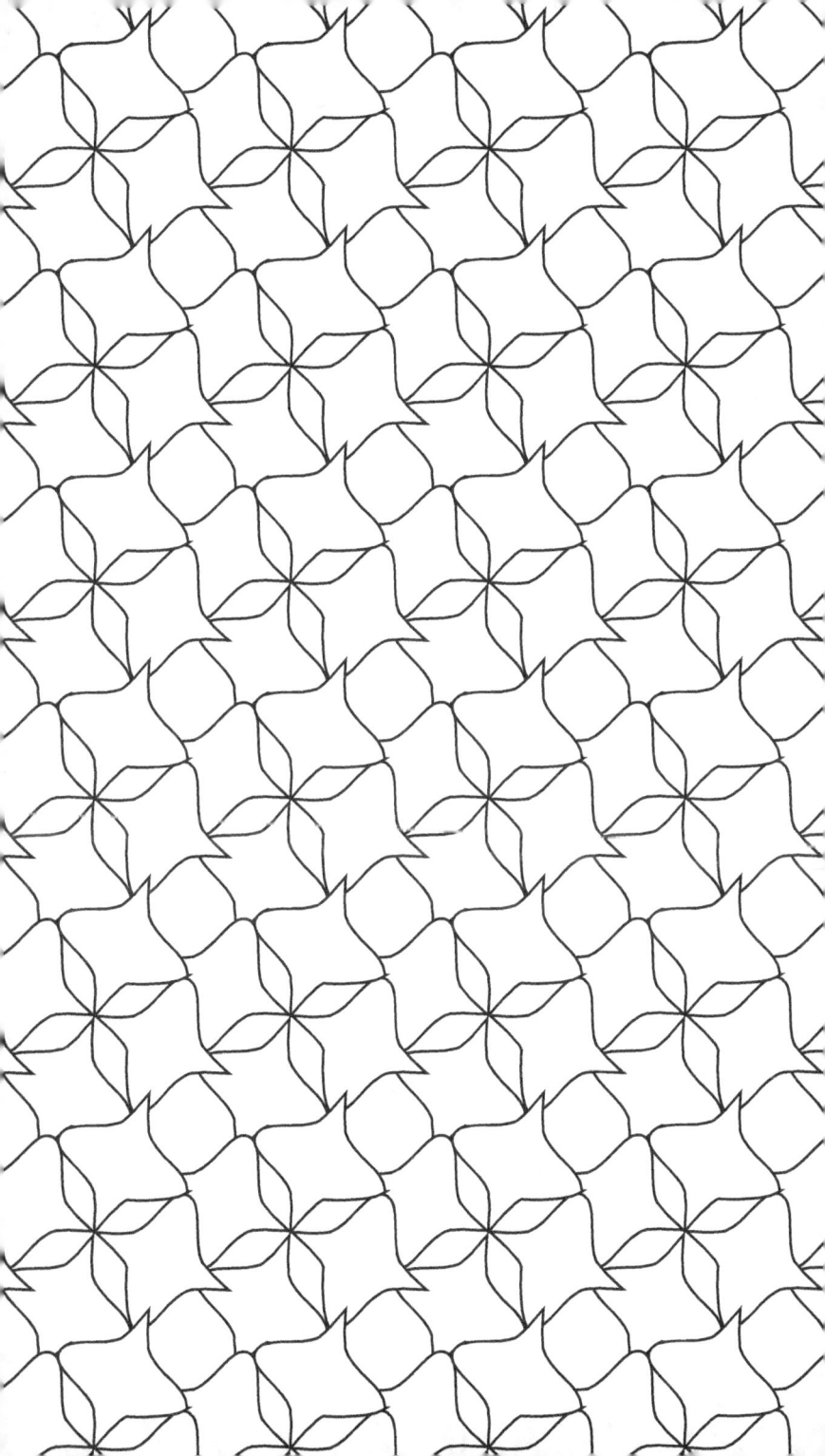

THE ESSENCE
OF ALL
BEAUTIFUL
ART,
ALL GREAT
ART IS
GRATITUDE.

FREDRICH NIETSCHE

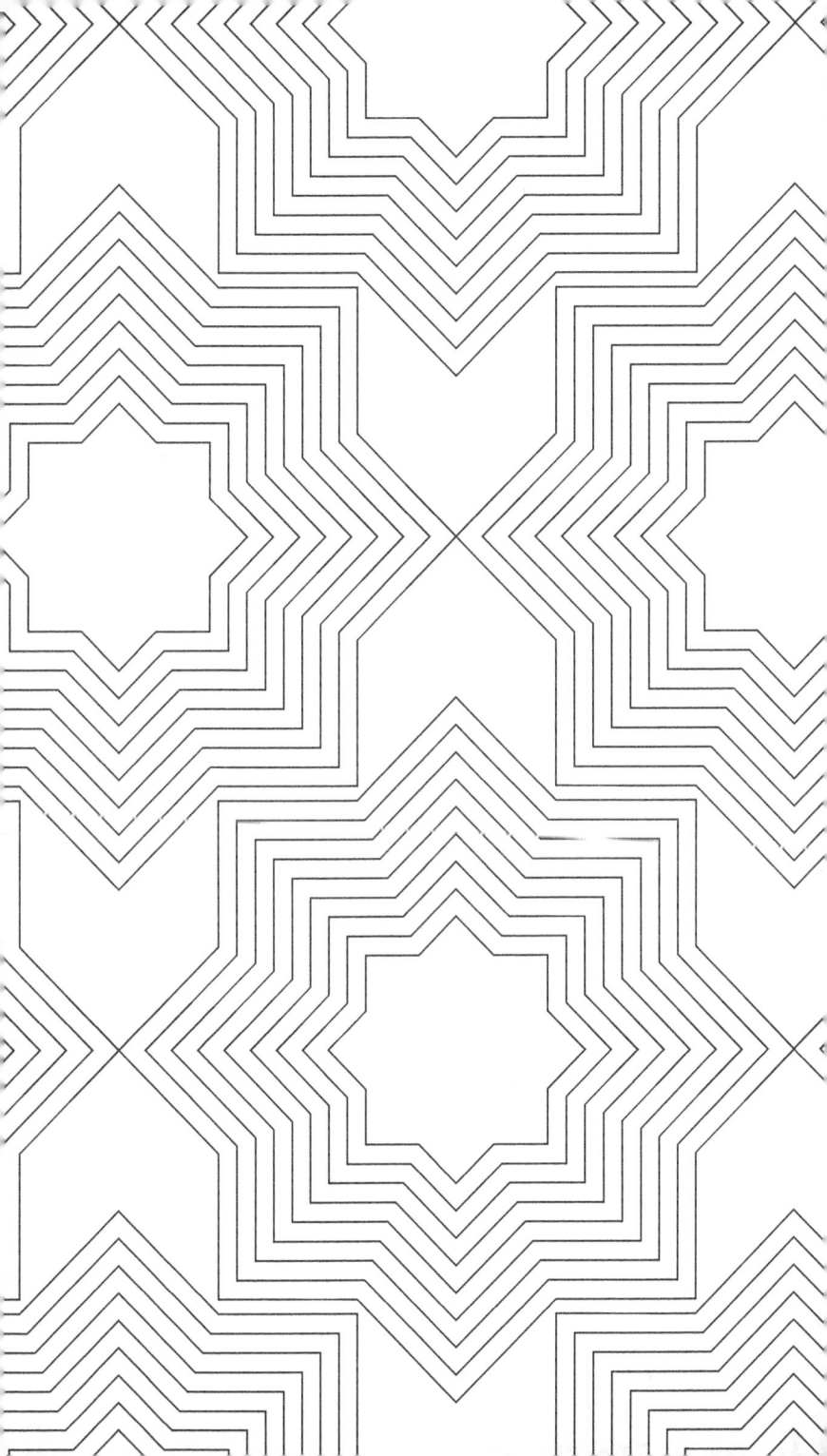

ART
IS NOT
WHAT
YOU SEE,
BUT WHAT
YOU MAKE
OTHERS
SEE.

EDGAR DEGAS

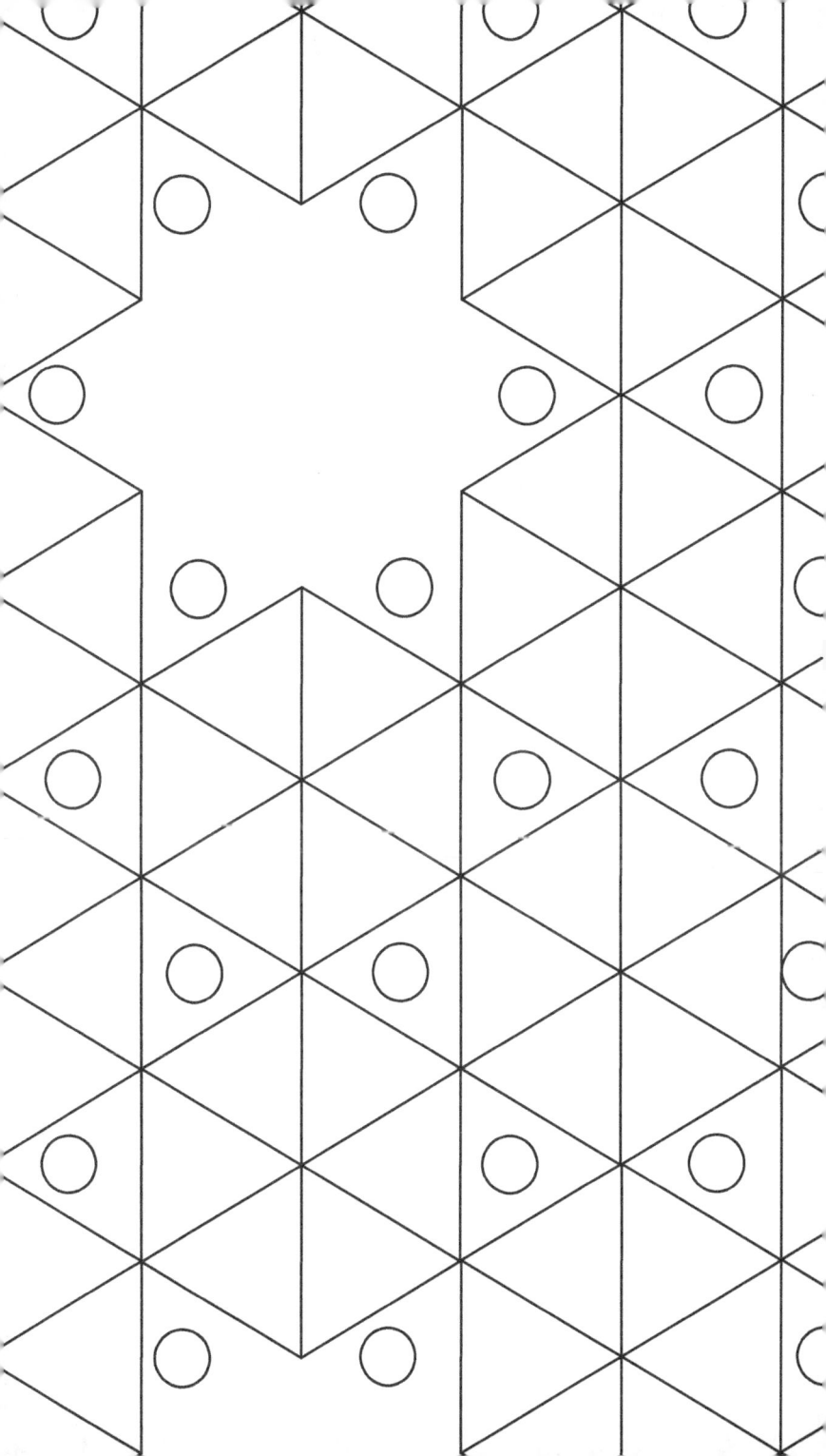

TO BE AN ARTIST IS TO BELIEVE IN LIFE.

HENRY MOORE

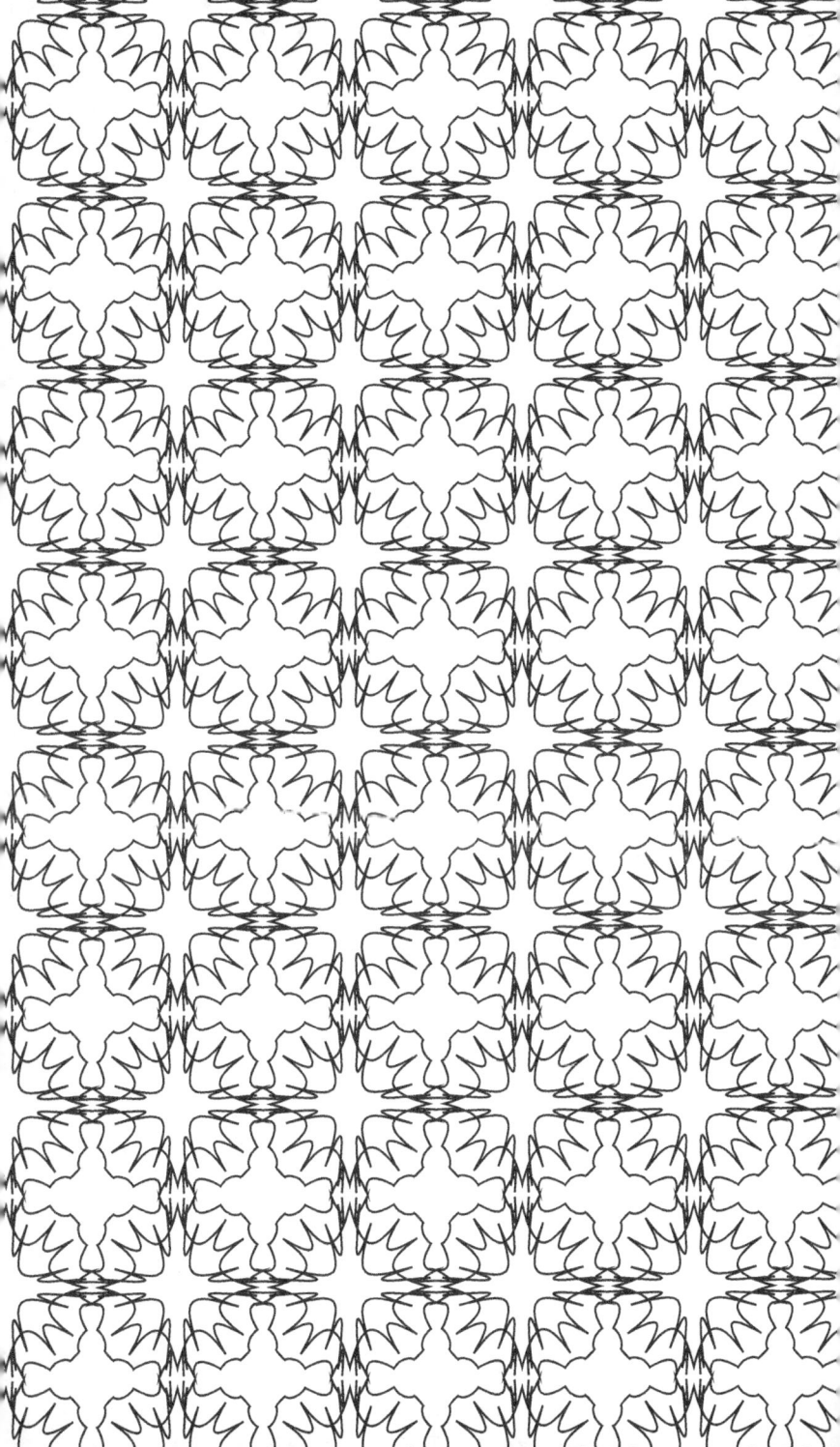

A WORK OF
ART IS A
SCREAM OF
FREEDOM.

CHRISTO

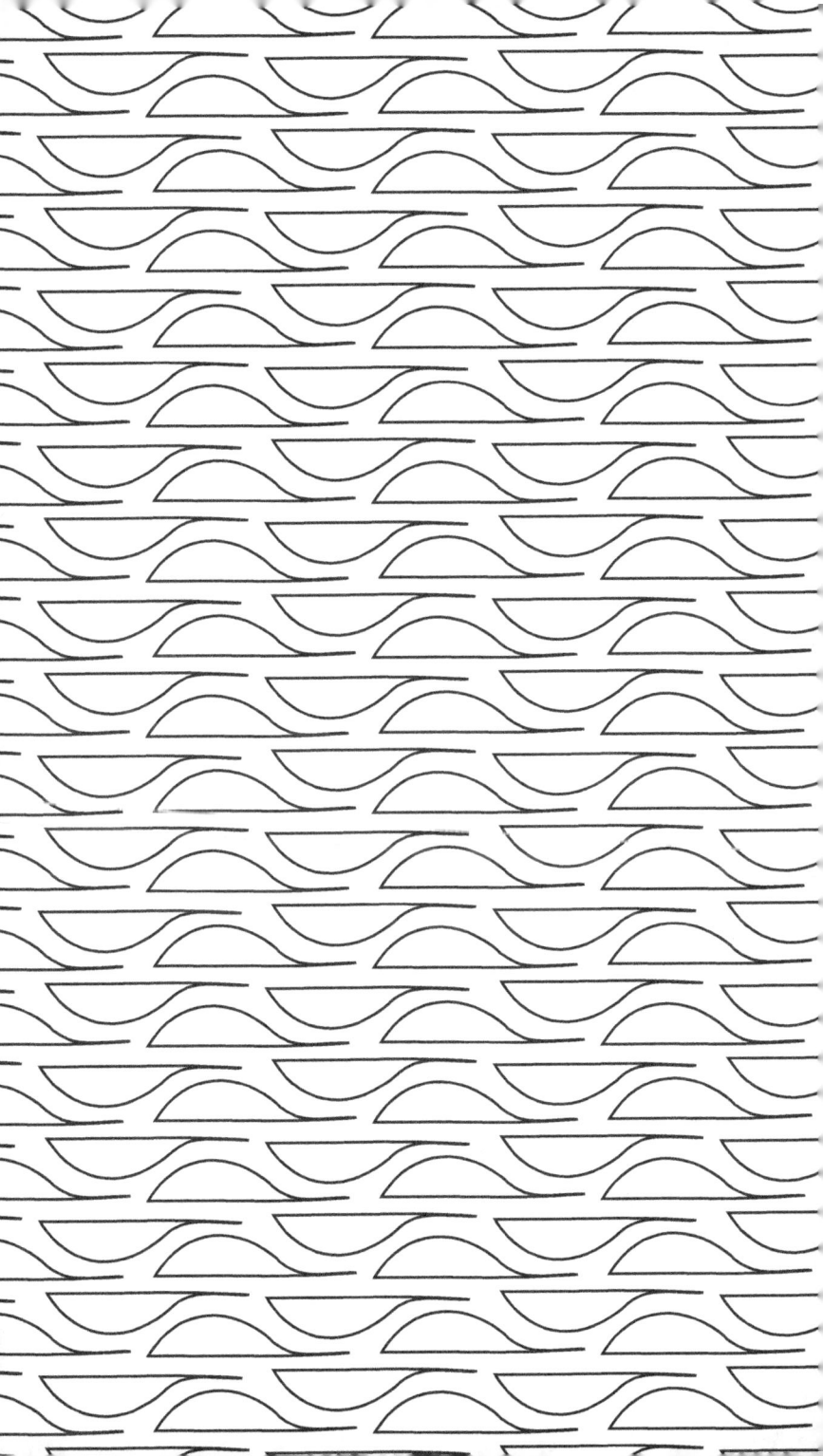

THE
"EARTH"
WITHOUT
"ART"
IS JUST
"EH"

UNKNOWN

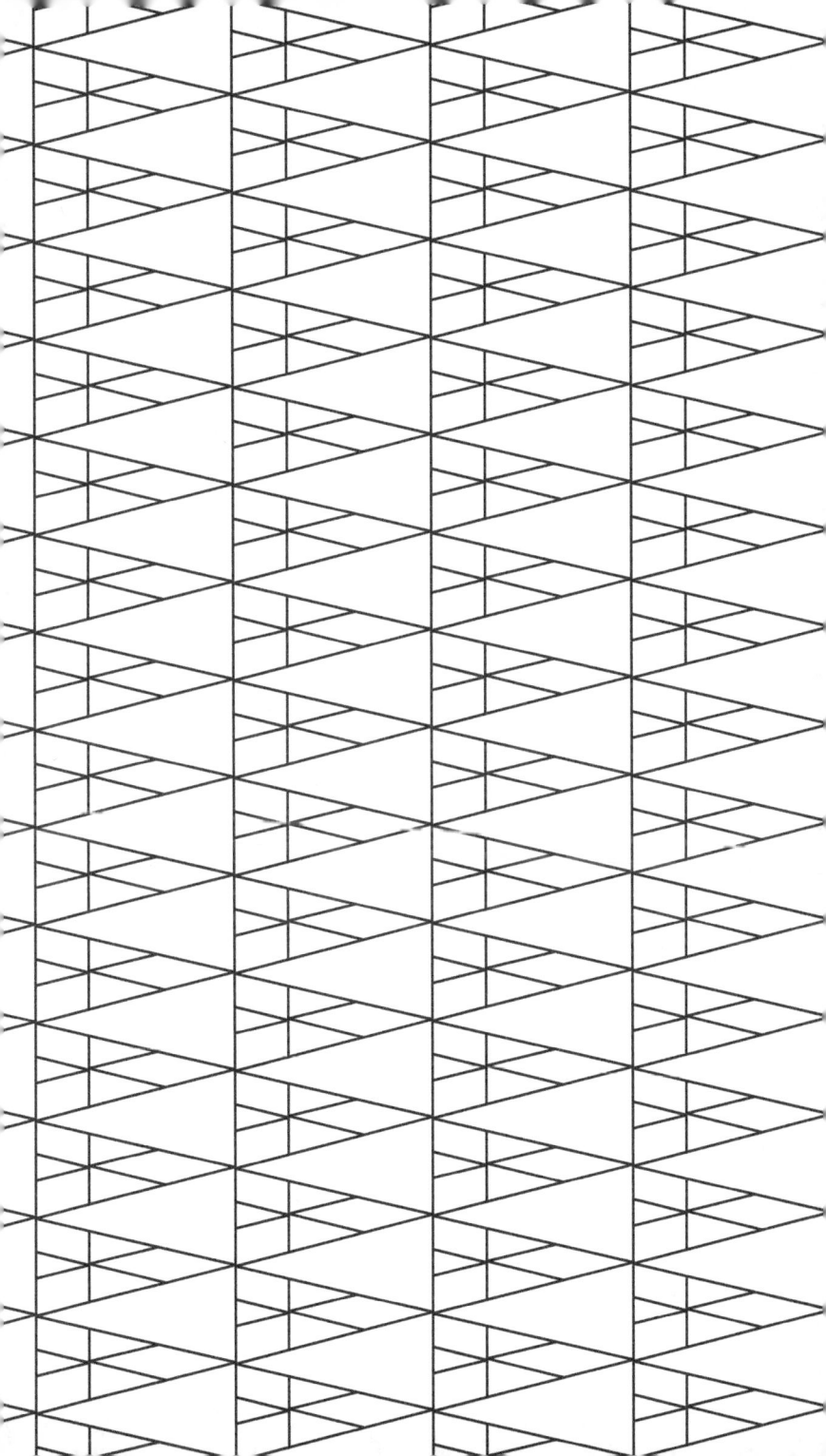

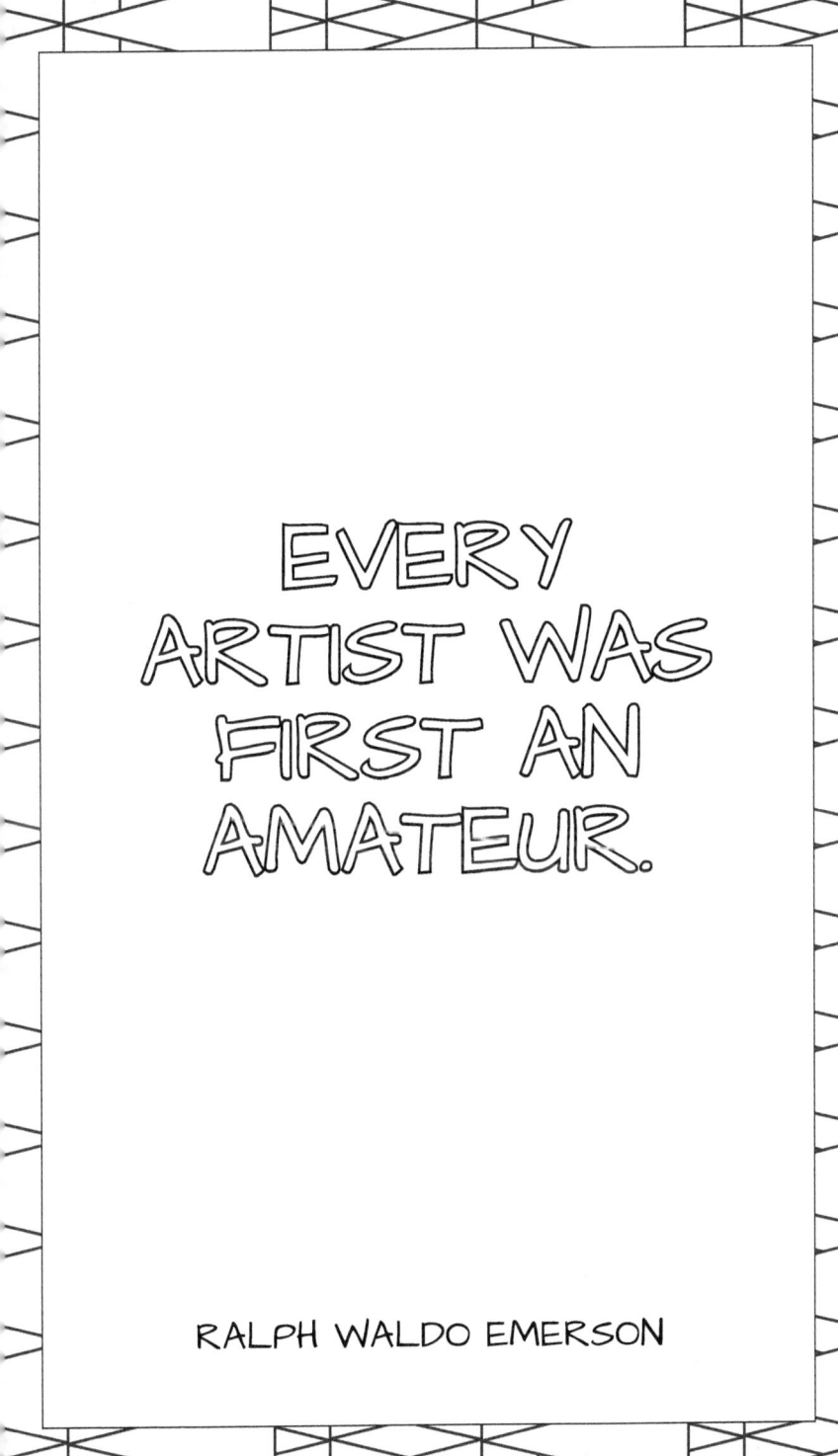

EVERY
ARTIST WAS
FIRST AN
AMATEUR.

RALPH WALDO EMERSON

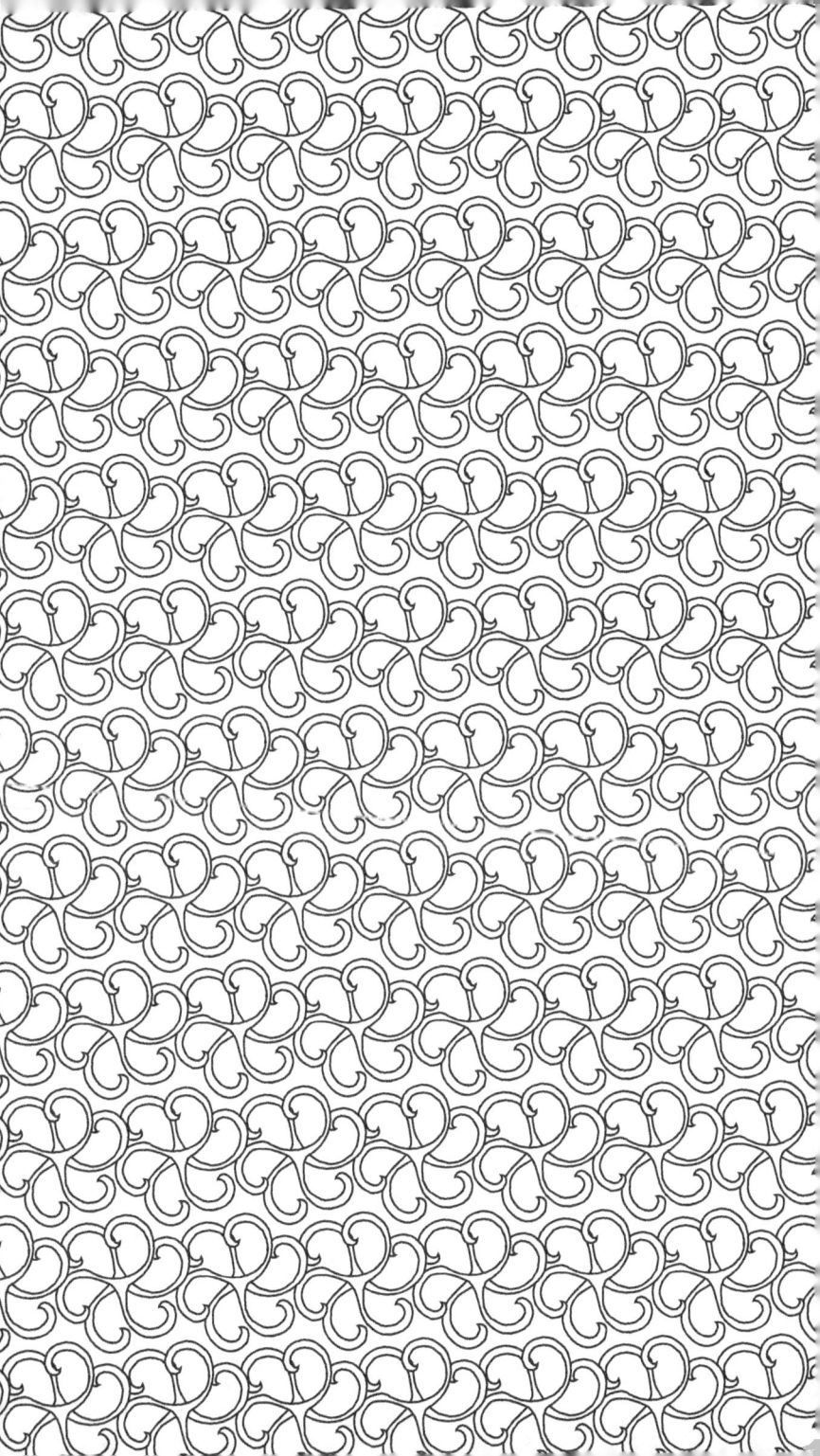

ART
SHOULD
COMFORT
THE DISTURBED
AND DISTURB
THE
COMFORTABLE.

CESAR CRUZ

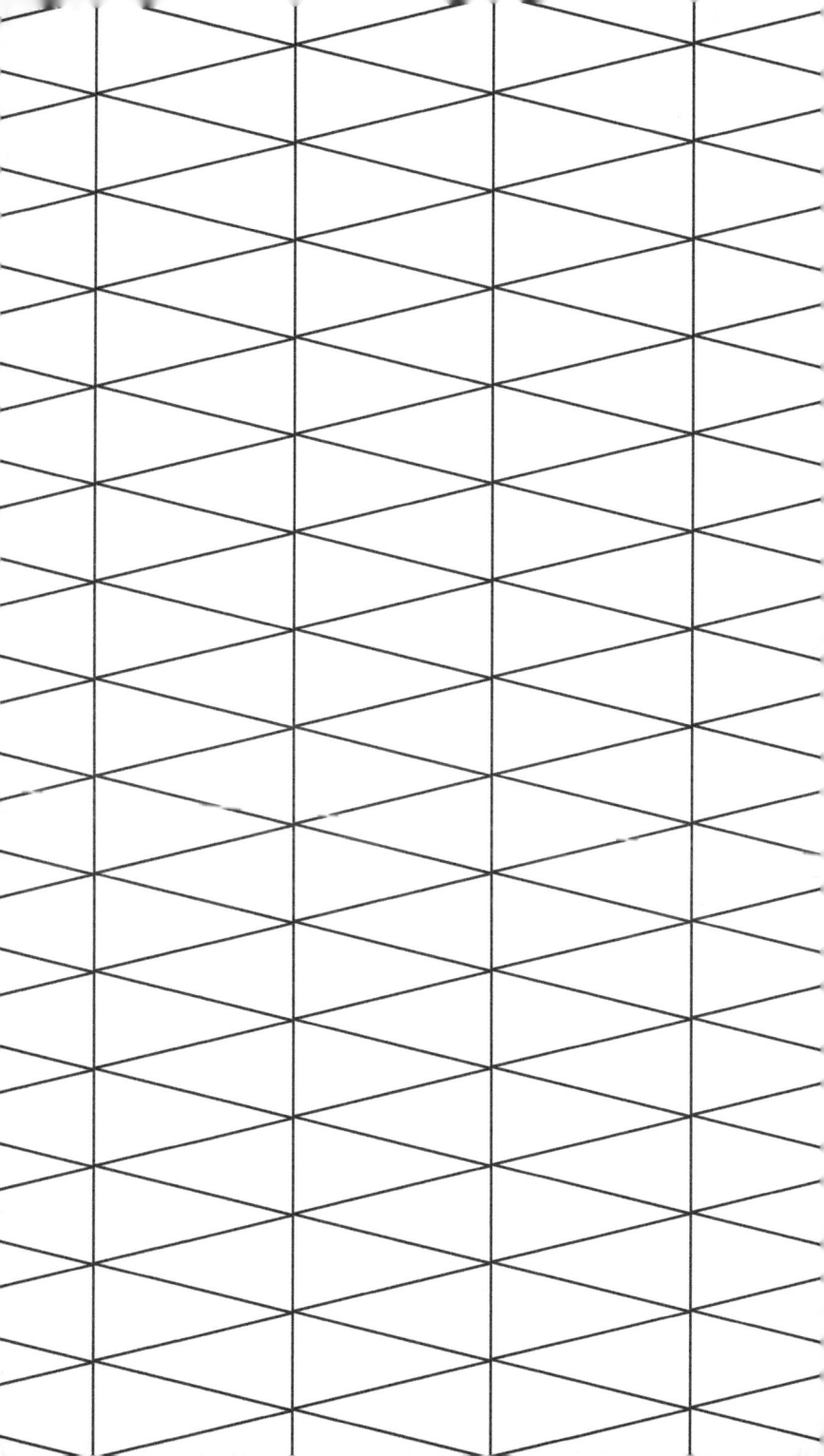

ART
IS NEVER
FINISHED,
ONLY
ABANDONNED.

LEONARDO DA VINCI

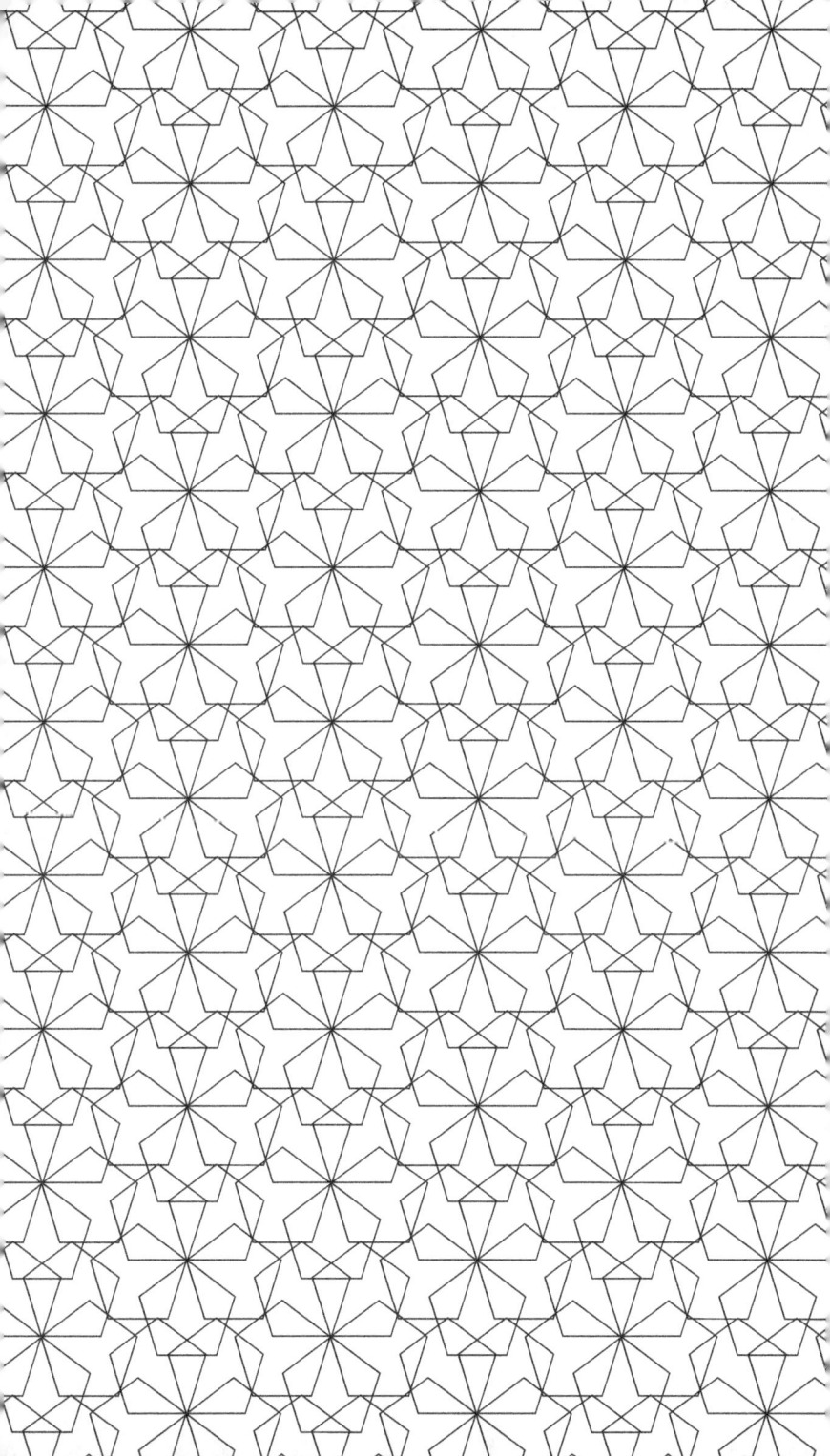

COLORING OUTSIDE THE LINE IS A FINE ART

KIM NANCE

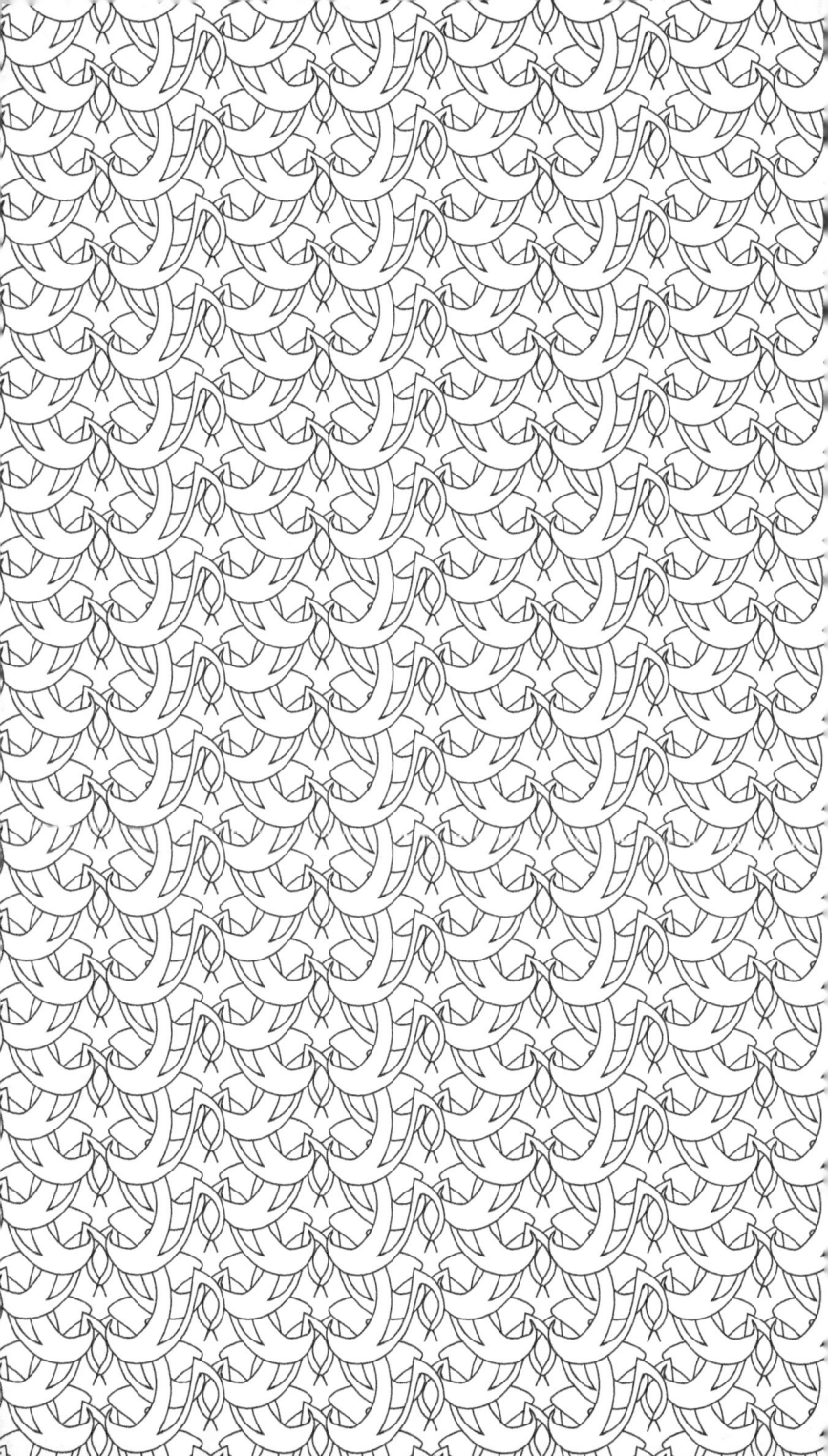

COLORS
ARE THE
SMILE
OF
NATURE

LEIGH HUNT

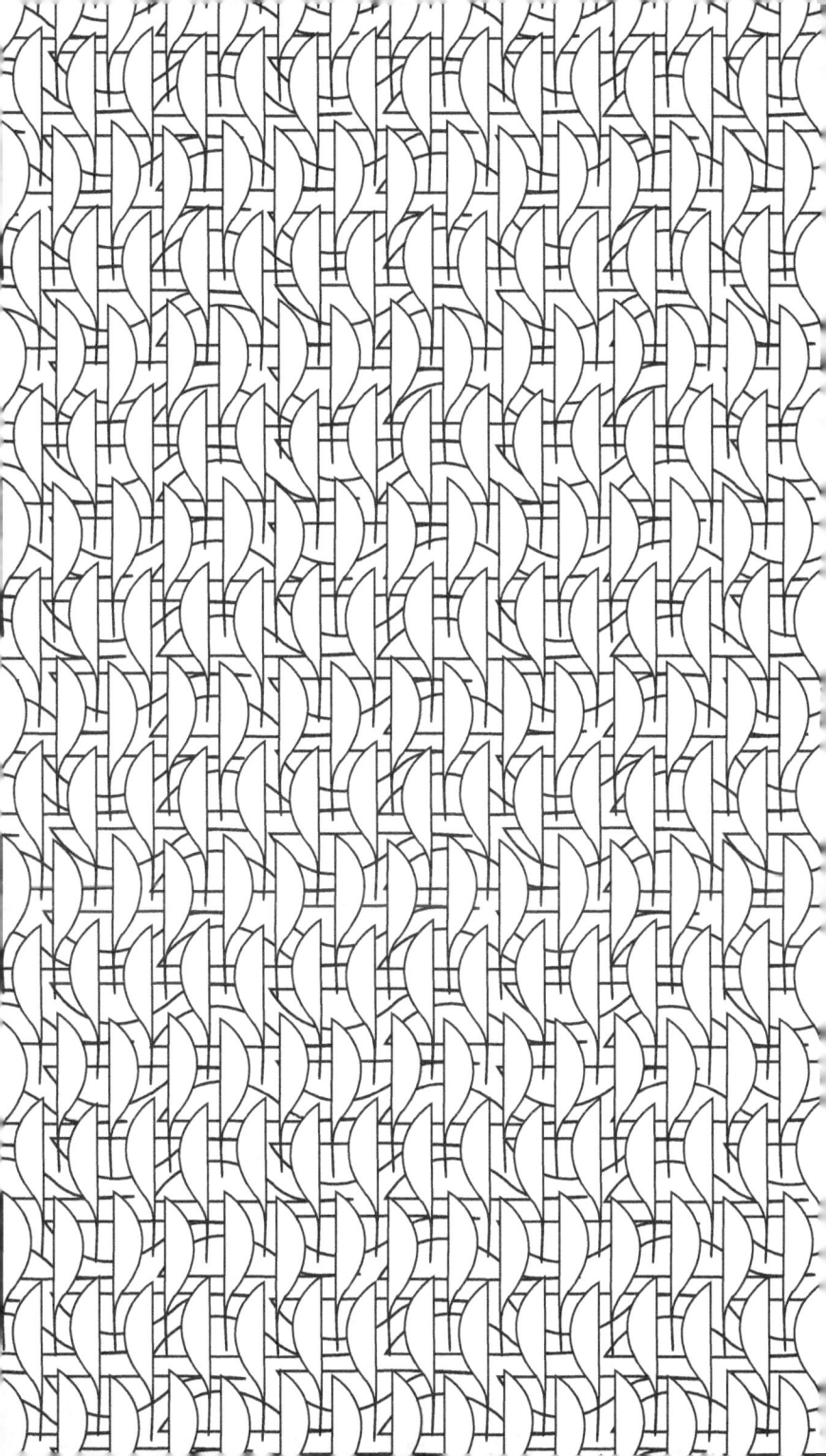

COLOR IS MY DAY-LONG OBSESSION, JOY AND TORMENT

CLAUDE MONET

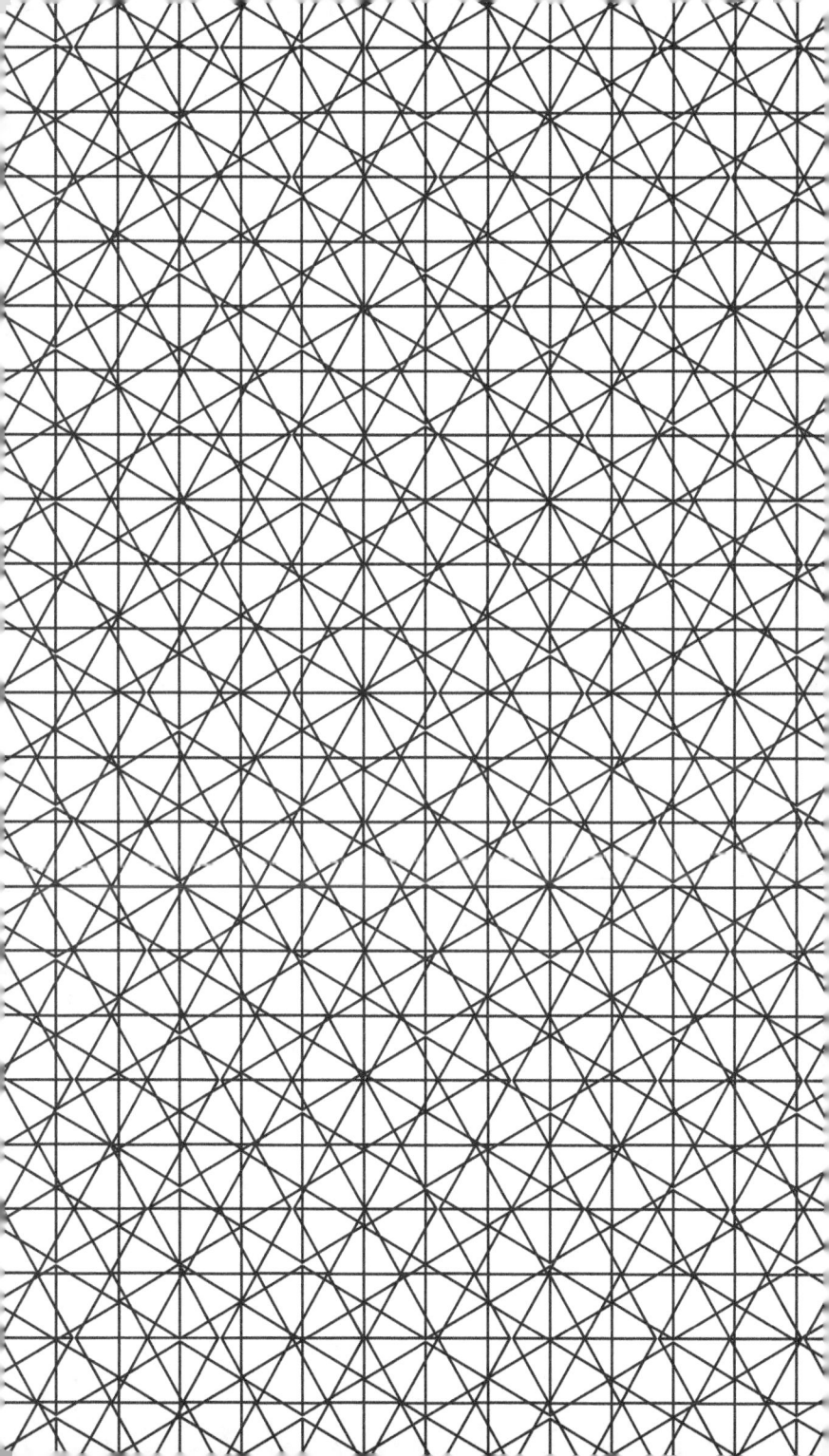

GIVE CRAYONS !

ADULTS ARE DISTURBINGLY IMPOVERISHED OF THESE MAGICAL DREAM STICKS !

DR. SUN WOLF

 Share your masterpieces on Instagram
@pagecoloring